NUTRITION AND THE MIND

By Gary Null, Ph. D.

FOUR WALLS EIGHT WINDOWS

New York § London

A Four Walls Eight Windows First Edition.

All rights reserved.

Printed in the United States of America.

Four Walls Eight Windows
39 W. 14th Street, #503
New York, N.Y. 10011

10 9 8 7 6 5 4 3 2 1

Interior design by Morgan Brilliant.

Library of Congress Cataloging-in-Publication Data

Null, Gary.
  Nutrition and the mind / by Gary Null.
  p. cm.
        Includes bibliographical references and index.
  ISBN 1-56858-021-5 : $14.95
  1. Mental illness—Nutritional aspects. 2. Orthomolecular therapy.
  3. Mental illness—Diet therapy. 4. Behavioral toxicology. I. Title.

RC455.4.N8N85 1995   94-46982
616.89'1—dc20   CIP

TABLE OF CONTENTS

Preface

It is estimated by the National Institute of Mental Health that more than 40 million Americans are affected by any one of a number of mental and emotional conditions that adversely affect the quality of their lives. These include depression, schizophrenia, bipolar disorder, dementia, and autism, as well as other conditions, which, while they may not fall strictly under the rubric of "mental illness," have a mental component, e.g., fatigue, insomnia, learning disabilities, attention deficit disorder, eating disorders, PMS, alcoholism, and aggressive behavior. When you consider that probably an additional 50 million people suffer from intermittent bouts of one or a number of these conditions, then you can see that close to one third of the entire American population is personally grappling with mental health concerns.

Yet despite the extent of mental disorders, the American medical establishment has paid little attention to causes, so intent are they on obtaining the relief of the symptoms of these conditions. Take alcoholism, for instance. There are dozens of studies showing that alcoholics are chronically deficient in certain essential nutrients. Other studies show that when these nutrients are given at optimal levels, the chemical imbalances that precipitate the craving for alcohol are diminished or eliminated, thus biochemically breaking the addictive response. One would think that the medical establishment would at least attempt to address the ramifications of these studies in the approaches to treatment that are currently favored. But they have not done so. Currently, many tens of billion dollars are being spent yearly on drug and alcohol treatments, of which the vast majority ignore nutrition-based approaches. Since few of the now-prevalent approaches have been shown to be successful, it is worrisome that nutrition-based approaches continue to be relegated to the margins. We need to look at the fact that when biochemical imbalances are corrected and chemical sensitivities addressed, the treatments work, and with a lack of relapse. This is the kind of cause-and-prevention oriented approach we should be encouraging, for alcoholism and other problems.

It is in an attempt to help encourage such an approach that I put together this book. In it, 25 of America's leading holistic physicians explore their experience in dealing with various mental health conditions, and patients describe their experience as well. I've interviewed nearly 500 individuals in depth—psychiatrists, psychologists, behaviorists, neuropsychoimmunologists, and environmental medicine experts, among others. Some of these people have particular areas of specialization, such as autism, alcoholism, or fatigue. By the way, fatigue, or lack of energy, is a condition that probably affects more people and yet receives less attention than any other. Fatigue—not just chronic fatigue syndrome, but simple fatigue—affects peoples' attitudes and behavior, and is a common factor in depression, bipolar disorder, and insomnia.

After interviewing the experts in a variety of fields, it was remarkable to see how many used similar treatment modalities—treatment with vitamin C or the B complex vitamins, for example—and to see also that their therapeutic approaches had certain elements in common, such as cleansing the body of toxins through diet, and rebalancing the body through the use of herbs, botanicals, nutrients, and proper diet. It should be noted that all of the treatment modalities mentioned in the following material have been proven successful.

In addition to interviewing hundreds of clinicians—and getting input from over 3,000 patients—I've reviewed thousands of articles and abstracts in scientific peer-reviewed journals in preparing this material. I've included summaries of some of these articles in an appendix to this book so that interested readers can see that, yes, we do have a scientific basis when we claim that nutritional deficiencies play a role in precipitating the biochemical imbalances that lead to a variety of conditions, and that, yes, nutritional treatment does have scientifically proven value in alleviating these conditions.

Concerning the scientific literature, we have an interesting phenomenon in America today. We have thousands of articles in peer-reviewed journals clearly demonstrating that nutrition will affect either the cause or treatment—or the prevention—of different diseases. It is estimated that up to 90 percent of all diseases could be eliminated if we understood the role that nutrition plays. Now that we have the evidence, the question is, why have the medical community, the educational community, and the media not advocated that we implement it?

One of the problems is that once a physician has been trained in a particular area of specialization in a particular way, for that physician to relinquish his or her mind-set and embrace a new paradigm of knowledge is not an easy process. Even with the best of intentions for their patients' well-being, doctors will continue to use modalities that have been outmoded, or that have been shown to be of no benefit, or that are actually harmful, for the simple reason that one uses what one knows. Examples abound: radical mastectomies, hysterectomies, Cesarean operations, coronary bypass operations, electroconvulsive therapy, and Thorazine. All have been associated with devastating side effects, high mortality rates, or chronic abuses, and yet are the preferred treatment modalities for many physicians. There exist nontoxic, successful alternatives to all of these that are being ignored by the medical establishment, although the scientific basis is now there to more than justify a fundamental change in treatment modalities toward nutrition-based approaches.

We must also consider the power and influence of the pharmaceutical industry and of the various medical technology industries. These would stand to lose a substantial part of the 1.3 trillion dollars, year in and year out, that our national sickness care system costs the American public. Were the public to change its perspective on the nature of acceptable treatment and begin demanding nontoxic therapies, that cash cow would be no more.

Despite the forces defending the medical status quo, change is happening. There are some physicians—albeit a relative handful out of the 600,000 in the U.S.—who are using the therapies referred to in this book. These physicians are revolutionizing American health care. There is also a growing segment of the public becoming aware of these nontoxic therapies. But the impact of these new forces is only just beginning to be felt in mainstream America.

This book will, I hope, greatly expand the reach of this new medicine. It was written with the idea of helping to ease the enormous costs of mental health care, both nationally and to individuals, both economically and emotionally, across the nation.

The answers are here. The challenge for the future rests in their implementation, which will require diligence on the part of the media, a focused legislative process, and a committed medical community, working in unison to see that these answers are given proper attention.

—Gary Null

NUTRITION AND THE MIND

INTRODUCTION:
THE PROMISE OF VITAMIN THERAPY
(ORTHOMOLECULAR PSYCHIATRY)

Orthomolecular medicine and orthomolecular psychiatry are now over a quarter of a century old, having started with Dr. Linus Pauling's 1968 article in *Science* Magazine called "Orthomolecular Psychiatry." As Dr. Philip Hodes explains, "'Orthomolecular' means the right amount of the right nutrients. . . . Thanks to Dr. Roger Williams's concept of 'biochemical individuality,' and Dr. Bernard Rimland's concept of 'toximolecular brains,' we found that many people with so-called mental illnesses, including schizophrenia, autism, depression, and manic-depression, can be helped, in a majority of cases. They must first clean the toxins out of the brain and then provide the brain with the right amounts of the right nutrients.

"Each person is biochemically individual," Dr. Hodes continues, "so the government standards for the minimum daily requirements of various nutrients actually have little if any bearing on the specific needs of any particular human being. What seems to be a mega-amount for one person is the precise amount necessary to keep another person healthy and sane."

1

Psychiatrist Michael Schachter says that most psychiatrists will consider the possibility of a chemical imbalance in the brain as well as any psychosocial factors. In the former case, they then immediately resort to using some kind of drug to try to right the balance, without looking into the possibility that there could be nutritional factors contributing to the patient's psychological state. "I explore possible imbalances in the body that could be caused by nutritional and other environmental, nonpsychosocial factors that might be playing a role in the development of psychological symptoms. For instance, they don't bother inquiring how much sugar a person is eating, or how much coffee someone is drinking. They do look at alcohol consumption, especially if it's excessive, but most psychiatrists are unaware that sometimes even small amounts can be a problem."

Whenever possible, Dr. Schachter prefers nutrition-based therapies. "I use nutritional substances or substances that are natural to the body, either food substances or accessory food factors—such as vitamins or minerals or amino acids—as the treatment of choice for a person's mental disorder. Sometimes the vitamins may be megadoses because a person may be what we call vitamin-dependent on a particular nutrient. For example, some children who are hyperactive or having learning disorders will respond to one vitamin, for instance vitamin B_1 (thiamine), and actually might get worse if you give them large doses of vitamin B_6. So treatment really has to be individualized. I try to find what seems to be most effective for that particular child's or adult's condition."

Hand in hand with the nutrition-based approach, Dr. Schachter looks closely at the clinical ecological factors: the foods in the person's current diet, the water he or she drinks, the air he or she breathes, any imbalances in the body, as well as any daily-life habits. "For example, I check for hormonal imbalances or subtle low-thyroid conditions, which are very common in depression. If these are treated, there will often be marked mood improvement. Calcium and magnesium deficiencies are very common as precipitators for anxiety in general or even panic attacks. By correcting some of these nutrient imbalances, you can reduce tremendously the chances of a person having panic attacks. Then, if everything else is not sufficient to bring about improvement, I would use psychotropic drugs if I had to, but I would try to keep them at the lowest possible dose and I would use nutrients and other dietary supplements to minimize their side effects."

In 1955, Dr. Abram Hoffer and several colleagues published a paper in which they showed that nicotinic acid lowered cholesterol levels but that you had to give 3,000 mg per day. This was a major step forward because it proved that you sometimes needed large amounts of a vitamin for a condition not known to be a vitamin deficiency disease. High blood cholesterol was not known to be a vitamin deficiency disease. The term "orthomolecular" was developed by Dr. Linus Pauling as presented in his paper in *Science* in 1968. It was based upon his recognition that certain vitamins are effective when they are used in large quantities.

At that time, the conventional wisdom was still that you used vitamins only in tiny amounts and you only needed them for the prevention of deficiency diseases, like scurvy or beriberi. A nutritionist accepted the fact that if you had scurvy you would eat oranges or you would take small quantities of vitamin C. As Dr. Hoffer puts it, "It was unheard of to give someone a thousand mg of vitamin C. If you suggested this they would throw up their hands in horror. The idea that you could use large quantities of vitamins to treat conditions, not just to prevent them, was a major step forward. In fact, it is considered a major paradigm change.

"This was the beginning of the contemporary model, which is that in certain cases you need large quantities of vitamins to treat conditions that are not assumed to be vitamin deficiencies. For example, in a recent Harvard study, over 100,000 subjects were given vitamin E. The study found a 40 percent reduction in their coronary rate. No one looks upon coronary disease as a vitamin deficiency and yet substantial quantities of vitamin E—they used 100 I.U. a day—are very effective. So we are now in a paradigm in which we use vitamins as treatment, not just as prevention."

Dr. Hoffer emphasizes this development in his clinical approach. "Orthomolecular psychiatry and medicine was the first major movement to adopt this treatment paradigm. What it means is that when we have a sick patient, we correct their diet. This is vital. I don't talk to any patient until we have spent some time on their diet. We also use any drugs that have to be used. If I have a schizophrenic patient I will use tranquilizers; if I have a depressed patient I will use antidepressants; if they're epileptic I'll use anticonvulsants; if they're suffering and in a lot of pain, I'll use analgesics. But that's not all. In addition to that we use the appropriate nutrients. It can be any one of the 20 or 30 nutrients currently in use. We combine them all. When the patient begins to respond, we gradually withdraw the drugs until we are able to maintain them on the nutrients alone or on such a tiny amount that it doesn't interfere with their ability to function.

"Orthomolecular medicine is the appropriate use of molecules, nutrients, which are native to the body in the appropriate concentration at the appropriate time.

"I don't like the term 'alternative.' I think, rather, that we are going back to our historical roots. If you go back 100 years we had no treatment except nutritional treatment. For 2000 years the best doctors in the world always emphasized good nutrition, but over the past hundred years nutrition suddenly disappeared from medicine. We're just bringing it back again.

"And not just us. I'm delighted to say that the whole field of medicine is moving very, very quickly in this direction. If you've seen *The Wellness Letter* from Berkeley lately, there is a tremendous change in their attitude from a couple of years ago when they were totally against vitamins. Now they're extolling them to the skies. This is a fantastic change. I consider that we are the mainstream of medicine, even though most doctors don't yet recognize it. My colleagues in psychiatry are still ten years out of date. That's because of the natural conservatism of the profession combined with the fact that they have had the least training in biochemistry and physiology of all physicians and thus they are the least likely to look upon the body as a physiological organism. They look upon psychosocial problems as primary when, in fact, in many cases they are secondary. The American psychiatric establishment—including Canada, and including the National Institute of Mental Health—has taken a very strong position against the use of vitamins in psychiatry and have yet to reverse their position, because they're slow learners."

Dr. Garry Vickar believes that "Doctors have a tendency to close their minds to anything other than what they read in their literature." He suggests that there are ways to help your physician be a part of the healing process. "The name of the game is getting better. You can't make people want to treat you if you come at them and say, 'You guys are all wrong. You don't know what you're

have been great advances. On the toxicology side, since about 1968 or 1970 I have done a screening test for toxins that we call the hair test. It is possible to screen every patient for mercury, lead, arsenic, aluminum, cadmium, nickel, and get an accurate picture of the environmental input into the individual's overall health. The test was, unfortunately, unfairly criticized by the AMA and is not used nearly as much as it should be. Those who are nickel-afflicted are likely to be more allergic. Nickel is a free-radical generator and a sensitizer of the first rank. People with nickel-tainted hair tend to have nickel in their dental alloys or fillings. Nickel is even more sinister than the more well-publicized mercury, which is also a sensitizer. There is nickel in the braces that kids wear, and they can pick up nickel in their systems that way.

"How do we test today if a person is, for example, sensitive to apples or to the sprays that are used on them, that is, to pesticides or chemicals? Some immunology labs are now offering remarkably helpful testing for chemical sensitivities for a relatively low cost. For about $200 you can get tested for seven or eight of the major solvents and chemicals, such as benzene and others that people haven't heard too much about. There are also plans to include the dioxins in this screening. These tests are a very helpful marker for environmental exposure. In addition, IGG4 and IGE testing can be done in tandem, in which a person is tested for a sample of food, chemical, and inhalant allergies by identifying antibody responses in the blood tests on an automated basis, thus bringing the price way down. These tests make it possible to get a powerful overview of toxicities and allergic responses inside a particular patient.

"Doctors who don't test their patients for toxicities and allergens are getting a limited view of their patients," Dr. Kunin concludes. "This can lead them to rely on treating symptoms with major tranquilizers, antihistamines, or other nonspecific therapies, rather than treating the source of an individual patient's problems."

Paying for the Care

According to Dr. Vickar, information about orthomolecular psychiatry is available to people who seek it out. But once the question becomes affording the treatment, there are obstacles. "Health care has become a political and economic issue. If you are bound by the restrictions of the standard insurance industry policy, you're going to have one devil of a time finding places to get this treatment covered. If you want to get into any kind of alternative health care program, you have to go outside of your regular health care.

"For the average individual—which includes most of us who have to buy health insurance—most insurance will barely cover psychiatric treatment to begin with, and most insurance certainly won't routinely cover the use of vitamins and mineral supplements, which can become quite expensive. It's not a matter of going out from time to time to buy a One-a-Day pill. You have to be using a large enough amount of vitamins to have a pharmacologic effect. You're talking about unreimbursible expenses for many people, so it becomes very expensive.

"There are areas in the country where people will be given greater access to complementary medicine. Perhaps California has that kind of mind-set where people think nothing of it. Complementary medicine is more limited in other parts of the country.

"We also have the problem that some products are no longer

available, for instance tryptophan, which was, and still is, I believe, a marvelous substance for people with mood disorders, alcoholism, and histories of drug abuse. It's off the market in the United States. The FDA has forbidden its use, on account of the appearance at one point of a tainted batch of the substance, even though the tainted tryptophan was isolated to a specific lab in Japan.

"I think removing tryptophan from the marketplace has been disastrous for many, many patients because it removed a valuable, safe treatment. It certainly affected a large number of mood disorder patients, many of whom were sleeping fine with the help of tryptophan."

Another barrier to the inclusion of orthomolecular psychiatry by standard insurance has been the paucity of double-blind studies. The money to fund such studies is not forthcoming, since there tends to be far less profit in vitamin therapies than in drug therapies. As Dr. Vickar notes, "Abram Hoffer did the very first double-blind study in psychiatry and then they criticized him for not having done double-blind studies!"

DISORDERS OF MOOD OR BEHAVIOR

1. Alcoholism

According to Dr. Robert Atkins, alcoholism is so tied in with carbohydrate metabolism that it is fair to say they are "genetically superimposable." In other words, it is possible to understand alcoholism in terms of carbohydrate metabolism alone. This is an extremely radical assertion, but one that lends important insight into a problem that plagues our society. "I have seen families in which half of the members were alcoholics and the other half were sugarholics," says Dr. Atkins. "And you could switch them over. You could probably make alcoholics of the people that were addicted to sugar, and it is well known that when alcoholics go through a psychologically based program, and not a biochemically based program, they have a tendency to become sugar addicts." In fact, it is unusual for ex-alcoholics *not* to become sugar addicts. More commonly, individuals replace one addiction for the other. As Atkins notes: "Unless people get the clue that there is a connection between alcoholism and sugar addiction, they will just go from one to another and will not feel any better. The phrase 'dry drunks' refers to what happens to alcoholics that start switching to sugar

13

instead of getting on a diet in which all the simple sugars are eliminated."

Clearly, in such situations nutritional awareness can make all the difference and Dr. Atkins considers it a necessary component of any successful alcoholism program: "Of course, nutritional support is also important. Minerals, such as chromium, zinc, and manganese, are all very important in regulating this sort of problem. Dr. Abram Hoffer also believes in the nutritional approach: "The general regimen that orthomolecular medicine uses for alcohol addiction (as with depression, schizophrenia, and a number of other mental disorders) is to pay careful attention to nutrition and the use of the right supplements.

"The first order of business," Dr. Hoffer continues, "is to make sure that the individual's basic diet is optimal. We do that by trying to take away most of the additives in food he or she eats on a daily basis. It is impossible to get them all out, but we try to do the best we can. One of the best simple rules is to put the patient on a sugar-free diet, because almost all foods that contain sugar contain a large variety of other chemicals. By avoiding sugar you will cut out most additives, by about 80 or 90 percent. Since we are all individuals, and many of us have food allergies and can't tolerate large quantities of carbohydrates or protein, for example, each one of us has to develop a diet that is optimal for ourselves.

"Second, we add in the supplements that are right for this particular individual. Many of us have been so deprived of these proper supplements over our lifetime that, even with a very good diet, we cannot regain our health. That's why we need supplements. This is where the treatment differs markedly from person to person (and depending upon whether someone is being treated for alcoholism, or a mental illness such as depression or schizophrenia). So while the dietary regimen is largely the same for all—avoid sugar and any foods that make you sick— supplements are determined on a case-by-case basis.

"For alcoholism the basic treatment starts with Alcoholics Anonymous. Bill W., the cofounder of Alcoholics Anonymous, first showed that when you added niacin to the treatment of alcoholism you got a major response that you did not see before. Today, there are a large number of very good alcoholism treatment programs in the United States, where they depend primarily on a combination of the type of nutrition that I have just referred to, the use of the right supplements, and the use of AA and other social aids to help these patients get well."

"Bob:" A Personal Account of Alcoholism

"I am a recovered alcoholic. It's been about seven years that I've been off alcohol. At first, I ate a lot of sugar in cakes and things like that. One of the psychological-emotional components of my behavior was that I always had a very difficult time getting started in the morning. The first thing I would think about when I got up was what I was going to eat, which usually included cereal with sugar, a pastry, and sugar-laden coffee. There has been a slow, progressive bettering of my diet, but there has still always been the sugar craving. Sometimes I would be able to get away from it for a week or two weeks, but it would always creep back in.

"Recently, I completed a seven-day fast and a colonic cleansing and I found that after that cleansing

process the craving pretty much disappeared. Also, I wake up in the morning feeling rather alert, and I don't have this compulsion to eat sweets. I think that because I am staying away from sugar, I generally am having better days psychologically."

2. Alzheimer's Disease

As the life expectancy of both men and women continues to increase, Alzheimer's disease, an only partially understood illness involving deterioration of brain matter and loss of brain function, has become an issue for increasing numbers of people. And yet, as the work of gerontologist Dr. Roy L. Walford, among others, has shown, it is possible to age in years while remaining functionally younger through enhanced nutrition and a diet that is somewhat different from the typical Western diet relying heavily on meat, dairy products, processed foods, and heaping servings. His most recent book, *The Anti-Aging Plan*, takes as its starting point the diet developed inside Biosphere 2 and adapts it to the less rigid daily-life habits of Americans, to come up with a low-calorie life-style that appears manageable and satisfying. In studies in mice, nutrient-rich caloric limitation diets largely eliminated age-related slowdown in rate of learning and in memory utilization.

Dr. Philip Hodes has developed a 14-step checklist of approaches he has found helpful in the treatment of Alzheimer's patients:

1. Avoid or eliminate any sources of aluminum exposure: aluminum cookware, utensils, or foil, underarm deodorants; drinking water and any juices and drinks packaged in aluminum-lined cartons. Cut out those vitamins as well as bottled water packaged in bottles with aluminum across the top.

2. Undergo a brain and body detoxification program, which should include a supervised fast. "Now don't attempt to detoxify on your own," Dr. Hodes warns. "You must have holistic physicians or practitioners who are knowledgeable, competent, and experienced in these practices, because if you attempt it on your own you may come up with some upsetting surprises."

Raw juice therapy helps flush out the toxins and supplies enzymes as well as raw vitamins and minerals. Colonic irrigation will help clean out the colon of years of accumulated putrefaction and helps the body function properly. Drinking distilled water, at least in the beginning or for part of the treatment, is also beneficial, along with the use of herbal noncaffeinated teas.

3. Have a practitioner of biological dentistry remove, in proper sequence, your silver-mercury dental amalgam fillings from your teeth. Tom Warren, who wrote *Beating Alzheimer's*, emphasized the importance of this procedure.

4. Bio-oxidative therapies are very effective in bringing oxygen into the brain to increase the individual's ability to think. We live in an external environment with only 19 percent oxygen, when it should contain 38 percent oxygen, so we all suffer from

oxygen insufficiency. Bio-oxidative therapies include hyperbaric oxygen chamber therapy, ozone therapy, and hydrogen peroxide therapy, among others. Also, superoxide dismutase, dimethylglycine, organic-germanium-132, glutathione peroxidase, homozone, vitamin E, aerobic exercising, and deep breathing in a relatively pure environment can be helpful. The herbs gingko biloba and butcher's broom are very beneficial.

5. The antioxidants, which work on the brain, are beneficial also. They include: vitamin A, beta carotene, thiamine hydrochloride, riboflavin, niacinamide, pantothenic acid, pyridoxine, B_{12}, folic acid, para-amino-benzoic acid (PABA), biotin, choline and inositol, vitamin E, vitamin C, vitamin P, the bioflavinoids (such as quercetin, hesperiden and pycnogenol), vitamin N, acetyl cysteine, acetyl carnitine, the sulfur-containing amino acids L-cysteine and L-methionine, and the enzymes such as co-enzyme Q10, bromelain, papain and pancreatic enzymes.

6. EDTA chelation therapy, performed intravenously, is very good for removing the heavy toxic metals, which include lead, cadmium, arsenic, nickel, copper, iron, mercury, and aluminum. A special chelating agent, desoxyferramine, works well, specifically as an aluminum-chelating agent.

7. Homeopathic remedies will also remove aluminum from the body and the brain, according to Dr. Hodes. "Then you have to take orthomolecular nutritional therapy, intravenously or with intramuscular

shots, along with oral supplements of all the nutrients."

8. Dr. Hodes credits clinical ecologists with having made a major contribution in the treatment of people with Alzheimer's disease when they recognized the importance of four to five day diversified food-rotation diets. In a food-rotation diet, you eat a variety of foods and no one food more than once or twice a week— thus eliminating the food allergens to which you are generally "addicted." The rotation diet also lightens the load on your immune system. You should also eliminate alcohol, caffeine, tobacco, sugar, and foods that are refined, processed, or filled with chemicals and artificial colorings and dyes. Replace them with natural, organically grown, pesticide-free wholesome and whole foods.

9. Biomagnetic and electromagnetic pulse therapies are also valuable. Diapulse, magnatherm, biofeedback, acupuncture, and ear acupuncture (auricular therapy) can also be tried.

10. Dr. Hodes also notes the existence of several other, less widespread approaches that are available, involving nutrient substances that increase brain function: An Israeli egg yolk lecithin substance, AL721, which was originally used to give energy and reduce cholesterol in elderly people, and also was used to combat HIV and AIDS, also helps the brain. You might try Dr. Ana Aslan's treatment called Gerovital (GH3) and live cell therapy, which are illegal in America but available in certain other countries. There is also something called super-triple-phosphatidylcholine.

Dr. Hodes adds: "There are supplement companies which manufacture brain formulas, which are composed of various amino acids, enzymes, vitamins, minerals, and herbs. Niacin, or vitamin B_3, is helpful because it opens up the blood vessels and brings nutrients, blood, oxygen, and other nutrients to the brain. Mineral baths, consisting of sodium, potassium, and magnesium, which seep into our bodies through the pores of the skin, are also helpful."

11. "Herbal remedies are also beneficial: Schussler cell salts, Bach flower remedies, and homeopathic remedies."

12. "Developmental/behavioral optometric vision therapy for improved visualization, perception, cognition, and memory efficiency."

13. "Cranial, sacro occipital technic, applied kinesiology, and network chiropractic and osteopathic care will improve the efficiency of the flow of the nerve supply and increase oxygen and blood carrying nutrients to the brain."

14. Finally, Dr. Hodes maintains: "Since the brain of an Alzheimer's patient shrinks, we have to rehydrate it with pure water, eight to ten glasses daily. It takes about six months to compensate for the shrinkage."

Dr. Michael Schachter describes his approach in dealing with Alzheimer's patients showing signs of senile dementia: "In the case of dementia, my approach is to see whether there are some nutrients that the person may need. Some people have improved quite a bit on a program in which they received injectable B vitamins and magnesium. Some of these elderly people have difficulty absorbing vitamins and minerals simply because of long-term chronic deficiencies, so an injectable program becomes very helpful.

"One of the first things I do is give them a trial of some vitamins and minerals by injection and often that will be very helpful to the patient. In addition, I have been using disodium-magnesium EDTA chelation therapy because by using disodium EDTA with magnesium we find that we're able to reverse some of the aging processes by removing calcium from soft tissues, where it doesn't belong, and trying to get it back into the bone, where it does belong. The chelation process, which is an intravenous treatment, will help with soft tissue decalcification, in addition to removing heavy metals.

"There is some research relating aluminum toxicity to Alzheimer's disease," Dr. Schachter adds. "Dr. Crapper McClaughlin has done some work in Canada, and we have been doing some work recently too, with patients who suffer from dementia using another chelating agent called Deferroxamine or Desferal, which is primarily useful in removing iron and aluminum—but not calcium—from the body. Usually, dementia is a one-way street; people tend to get worse and worse. By using this chelation process, some patients have at least had their dementia process slowed down or stopped for awhile. Some patients have even improved a little using a combination program of supplements, a good diet, and the removal of some of these heavy metals with chelating agents."

Dr. Hodes recommends the following books to obtain a more comprehensive picture of Alzheimer's disease and its treatment: Dr. Michael Weiner's *Reducing the Risks of Alzheimer's* (Stein and Day, 1987); Drs. Abram Hoffer and Morton Walker's *Smart Nutrients: A Guide to Nutrients that can Prevent and Reverse Senility* (Avery, 1994) and *Nutrients to Age Without Senility* (Keats,

1980); Ross Pelton's *Mind Food and Smart Pills: Nutrients and Drugs that Increase Intelligence and Prevent Brain Aging* (T&R, 1986); Tom Warren's *Beating Alzheimer's: The Case for Unlocking Brain Disease, Alzheimer's to Schizophrenia and Other Chronic Diseases* (Washington, 1988).

3. *Anxiety Disorders*

Anxiety disorders, including agoraphobia, claustrophobia, panic attacks, etc. often occur in people with prominent allergies. In many cases there is also a diet-related element relating to poor diet and/or poor absorption in the colon. Programs that address what are otherwise usually considered psychological and/ or biochemical problems *nutritionally* have met with much success, as have treatments relying on naturally occurring substances.

According to Dr. Allan Spreen, anxiety disorders will respond to treatment by certain natural substances. The advantages of treatment with natural substances can be numerous and substantial: by freeing people from having to take more toxic medication, the holistic approach can also spare the patient the medication's side effects, as well as the extra expense. "Some amino acids, when given individually," says Dr. Spreen, "in some cases can be very effective in calming down the symptoms of anxiety disorders and panic attacks. For example, tryptophan, which is no longer available, was used as a sleeping agent, until there was a problem with some batches of it being contaminated, which caused a syndrome that wasn't related to the tryptophan but to the contaminant. Some doctors use tyrosine for depression and anxiety. The 'DL' form of phenylalanine is often used on a short-term basis for depression and can be very effective if given correctly. It can lessen anxiety and depression in people by giving them more of an 'up' mood. Phenylalanine is also an appetite suppressant for many people. If they're given correctly there seems to be no toxicity associated with amino acids and they're much cheaper than antidepressants or anti-anxiety prescription medications."

Dr. Walt Stoll has a different approach: "In my clinical experience, I have found that emotional disorders are often linked to the inability to completely break down proteins, during the digestive process, into their amino acids. Just three or four amino acids still hooked together (peptides), if they get through the intestinal lining, can stimulate the immune system to make antibodies against them. Since our body is also made up of peptides, hooked together to make proteins, these antibodies can attack *us*. To an antibody, a peptide is a peptide. It frequently doesn't matter whether the peptide came from outside the body or is a part of the body. Many of the chronic diseases, which presently are so baffling to the allopathic disease philosophy of conventional Western medicine, are now being found to be related to auto-immune processes.

"In addition," Dr. Stoll adds, "some of these peptides have been found to be identical to certain brain hormones (endorphins) that are associated with panic attacks, depression, manic depression, schizophrenia, and other conditions. In these cases—with more certain to be discovered—there is no need for the immune system to be involved; the effect is direct. The two first examples to be discovered were peptides from imperfectly digested casein (milk protein) and gluten (wheat protein). Of course, these are the two most commonly eaten foods in our culture!

"All of the mental states listed above are at least partially caused by brain chemistry abnormalities. Generally, I see patients who have already tried many different therapies. These patients come with stacks and stacks of records documenting that nothing seems to have worked in spite of every imaginable test having been done and every imaginable treatment having been tried. Psychoactive drugs have either worked poorly or have even caused the problem to worsen due to the side effects exceeding the benefits.

"Since every other conceivable cause has been ruled out by the time I get to see them, I am free to look for the things that have not been evaluated. One of the first things I look for is how well the lining of their intestinal tract protects them from their environment. I frequently find that either they don't have the normal bacterial balance in the colon or that they have gone beyond that stage to having candidiasis. Candida can only escape from our control if the normal bacteria are *not* in control. If candida has converted from the normal yeast form into the disease-causing fungal form, it further damages the lining so that the leakage of peptides is much greater.

"The greater the amount of peptide leakage, the more likely it is that the brain will interpret these protein particles as being identical to the endorphins it produces during panic attacks, depression, etc. This same leakage is responsible for the increasing sensitivities we see in patients who are sensitive to environmental substances other than foods. It is much simpler, in most cases, to correct the leakage than it is to eliminate the substance. But why not do both?

"Once the reason for the leakage is corrected, the patient usually sees dramatic improvement in a very short time. The antibodies involved only last for 72 hours. Once the leakage is stopped completely, symptoms lessen substantially in just a few days; and just reduction of the leakage helps. There are many patients today that have had that kind of experience. Not everyone's mental symptoms are caused by poorly digested food playing tricks on the brain. However, in my experience, it is the most commonly missed diagnosis and one that is relatively easy to resolve."

Dr. Michael Schachter emphasizes the importance of proper diet: "If you suffer from an anxiety disorder, you really need to clean up your diet. Getting off sugar and taking calcium and magnesium works. Also, balancing the stresses in your life, through meditation and other anxiety-reducing disciplines, is important."

4. Depression (Unipolar Disorder)

Depression is an extremely common problem in America; it affects people of all backgrounds. There are different degrees of depression, and its treatment has varied considerably according to trends in psychiatry, psychology, and psychopharmacology in recent decades, and depending on the severity of the condition.

Some of us call it "depression" when we are struck by feelings of mild sadness, of the kind that affect nearly everyone from time to time, often for no obvious reason we can put our fingers on. Certain times of the year are associated with mood lows, particularly at the beginning and end of winter, for example. Commonly, when someone close to us moves away or dies, or if we lose a job or have some other major disappointment, there's apt to be an even stronger mood reaction in almost everybody. There will be some sadness, perhaps some grief. Usually such periods of sadness or grief are of a limited duration. When they drag on for a longer period of time, or become much more profound, we may begin to speak of clinical depression.

The causes of depression may include genetic factors. As

Dr. William Goldwag explains, "These may be related to changes in the brain metabolism and the nervous system. We know about genetic factors through the action of certain drugs. We see what chemical changes take place. Obviously our individual chemistry is to a great extent determined by our genes. There are genes presently under investigation that are believed to be responsible for manic-depression-type illnesses, in which one fluctuates from hyperactivity to depression or limited activity. Every day another gene is being found that is responsible for some of these illnesses. The gene expresses itself through a change in chemistry."

It's common for depressed people to have a family history of depression. In addition to the genetic factor, such family histories may also be due to common environmental factors, shared experiences in depressed families, and poor eating habits that are passed on from one generation to another.

Environmental factors may play multiple roles among the causes of depression. For example, being raised in a family in which one or more people are depressed may often be associated with poor nutrition. As Dr. William Goldwag reminds us, "Just being exposed to depressed people can be an influence, since children learn how to behave by imitation. Also, family members are eating the same food, and if, for instance, the mother is depressed and cooking and serving her family, that food is apt to be sparse in nutrients since she is interested in just getting the meal over with and has difficulty finding enough energy to prepare it."

Being abused physically or verbally can be another factor that inhibits children of depressed parents. As a way of handling abuse the child may withdraw and become depressed and inactive as a defense against very harsh treatment from the parent.

As Dr. Doris Rapp describes it, mood disorders often lead

to battering of family members and intimates: "Husbands batter wives, wives batter husbands, they both batter the children, and boyfriends batter their girlfriends. Mother battering, I might add, is very common. Many of the children I treat beat, kick, bruise, bite, and pinch their mothers. When some individuals have typical allergies and environmental illness, if they have a mood problem, they can become nasty and irritable and angry. All I ask is, 'What did you eat, touch, and smell?' To help find the cause I try to discover whether the change in behavior occurs inside or outside, after eating, or after smelling a chemical. It might be a food, dust, mold, pollens, or chemicals, which not only affect the brain, but discrete areas of the brain. As a result, the allergen or food or chemical exposure might make you tired or, if it affects the frontal lobes, it might make you behave in an inappropriate way. It could affect the speech center of the brain so that you speak too rapidly, or unclearly, or stutter, or don't speak intelligently. It's just potluck as to what area of the brain or body will be affected when you are exposed to something to which you are allergic."

In the not-so-distant past, before drug therapy became popular, severe depression was treated through hospitalization, electroshock therapy, and even insulin shock therapy. Dr. Goldwag describes the reasoning behind such extreme measures: "The idea was that somehow or other when you shock the brain it shakes things up. A lot of the disturbed thought processes seemed to almost get blanked out, and you could sort of start all over again with an individual.

"Psychotherapy, of course, has always been popular," adds Dr. Goldwag. "That can range from just the presence of a close, supportive friend or relative to more in-depth treatment with a psychiatrist or psychologist."

Perhaps most importantly, when depression is relatively mild, there is much the individual can do on his or her own. According to Dr. Goldwag: "There are many, many things that individuals can do to help themselves. What we want to ask is, what can we do nutritionally and in other ways? What lifestyle factors are under our own control that we can manipulate in order to alleviate symptoms of depression or prevent them?"

Three of the most important areas where answers to that question can be found by the individual himself or herself are exercise, interaction with others, and nutrition.

Exercise is one of the most profound aids in the treatment of depression, according to Dr. Goldwag: "One of the major errors in the thinking of patients and therapists is the notion that in order to be active you have to feel better. This is exactly contrary to what we are recommending.

"We recommend that you *do* first, and then the feeling comes later. In other words, you must do what you have to do regardless of how you feel. This aids in feeling better. You can't wait until you feel good and then do something, because in depression that may take days, weeks, months, or even years. You want to accelerate the process.

"Those of us who exercise regularly have had days when we just didn't feel like it. That's the way depressed people feel about everything. They just don't feel like it. They don't have the energy, the motivation, the stimulation to go and do even the ordinary things. When it's severe, the person may not even have the will or desire to get out of bed in the morning.

"The exercise may consist of very, very simple things, like just getting out and walking, getting up and doing some simple movements, some mild calisthenics, any kind of physical movement that gets the body in action. For some people just getting out of bed and getting dressed is a big accomplishment. That may be the first step.

"It is important for depressed people to get up and get dressed. They should not walk around in the pajamas or nightgowns because this maintains that connection to the bed and the bed means inactivity. That's the thing you're trying to overcome. Exercise may take the form of walking, walking the dog perhaps, or going outside to do some simple gardening. These are all very important for overcoming that feeling of lassitude that is so characteristic of depression.

"Another benefit of exercise is a feeling of accomplishment. Even doing a little bit of exercise will make you feel more energized later on. Finishing an exercise routine, even one that's fatiguing, after a brief period of rest, will give you a feeling of revitalization, of energy, and a psychological feeling of accomplishment. It gives a feeling of, 'I've done it. It's completed.' For the depressed individual, the boost to self-esteem that this can give is important."

Dr. Goldwag also emphasizes interaction with others as an important step the depressed individual may attempt on his or her own: "The next step may involve doing some volunteer work, getting out and doing things for other people. This is very important in trying to get the depressed person's mind off himself or herself. Depressed people are continually negative. They have dark thoughts, guilt, sad feelings, grief, regrets. Such negative thoughts are characteristic of depression. You can't talk the depressed individual out of them or try to convince them otherwise, but you can distract them. Physical activity is one distraction. Doing things for other people is another. So getting the person involved in someone else's problems can be a very effective way of dealing with depressed individuals."

Then comes nutrition. It is surprising how often diet and nutrition are factors in depression, and how effective enhanced or improved nutrition can be in helping someone suffering from depression to improve their mood. As Dr. Goldwag says, "Nutrition is important in preventing depression and treating it. Often the quality of the diet suffers in depressed people. If the depression is profound, the individual doesn't even feel like eating. Depressed people who live alone or who are major providers or cooks in the house may not feel like preparing meals or even shopping. They're apt to restrict their nutrition to fast food or just anything to get eating over with." In many cases, weight loss is a symptom of severe depression. In many other cases, there is substantial weight gain.

As Dr. Goldwag notes, significant weight loss is likely to bring about "marked deprivation of the essential nutrients, including the amino acids needed to manufacture the proper proteins, as well as a deficiency in many vitamins and minerals. That in itself can then aggravate the depression."

Dr. Goldwag suggests straightforward solutions to at least some of the challenges associated with depression: "There are some simple ways to prepare food in advance so that the food has to be prepared less often. I recommend preparing a raw salad once a week. Certain fresh vegetables can be stored for quite a period in a refrigerator and will keep quite well. There are a whole variety to choose from: carrots, celery, radishes, cauliflower, broccoli, peppers, red cabbage, green onions, snow peas, string beans. These can all be cut up and mixed together. They can be stored in a plastic bag or sealed container. When mealtime comes, a person can take a handful of these vegetables and then perhaps add some other ones that don't keep as well, such as tomatoes or sprouts. You then have a fresh salad that is already prepared with a lot of important nutrients. This is just one way of having food prepared in advance. It's good for people who are depressed and don't have the energy to make a whole meal."

Dr. Goldwag believes that the B Complex Vitamins are especially important. "One of the major groups of vitamins to incorporate are from the B complex family. Years and years ago, when people suffered from severe vitamin deficiencies, some of the resultant diseases like pellagra and so forth were characterized by accompanying psychotic reactions. That is, the thinking process was the most obvious one to be affected by the vitamin deficiency. Simply providing the proper vitamin, in this case vitamin B_3 or niacin, was the treatment. It cleared up the psychosis.

"There's no doubt that brain function is very dependent upon nutrients like niacin and others, because when they're absent there is apt to be some very disturbed thinking. Depression is one of the symptoms that can occur with this.

"It is important to get all the B complex vitamins, since they work together. Thiamine, B_1, is important, as is riboflavin to a lesser extent. Another important one is B_6, pyridoxine. B_{12} is still another one that can affect the mental processes.

"Niacin is often used in much higher doses than the others in order to accomplish some of these changes. Niacin is a ubiquitous vitamin. It is being used greatly to help reduce cholesterol levels, to improve the good cholesterol and reduce the bad. The dosages being used are much greater than those used to simply overcome a deficiency."

The amino acid tryptophan can be another key substance in the treatment of depression, according to Dr. Goldwag. Tryptophan helps to raise the levels of a naturally occurring chemical in the brain called serotonin, which have been found to be abnormally now in depressed people. "We learned about serotonin from experiments in which certain drugs that preserve it from being destroyed in the brain seem to work as antidepressants. The theory is that whatever can supply or aid the serotonin factor will help depression. Some foods that contain tryptophan can act as antidepressants. It is found most abundantly in milk and turkey. Tryptophan used to be obtainable until the FDA took it off the market several years ago because there were some serious blood problems in people who took it. This was later tracked down to a contaminant; the problem was not due to the tryptophan itself. Unfortunately the FDA has been rather lax in not allowing it back on the market again. Increasing the intake of milk and turkey are at least two ways of getting tryptophan."

At the same time, there are plenty of foods that should be avoided. Fast foods can affect mental symptoms by causing blood sugar abnormalities. People who tend to hypoglycemia or low blood sugar patterns should avoid eating too many simple carbohydrates, such as candy bars, which are converted very rapidly to sugar in the blood. As Dr. Goldwag says, "Simple carbohydrate foods temporarily raise the blood sugar, but then they drop it to a very low level several hours later, resulting in depression. This encourages the individual to repeat the cycle of taking sugar or some simple carbohydrate that's converted to sugar in order to feel that high again. This constant seesaw from high to low mood can account for many episodes of depression in individuals."

Both alcoholics and chronic dieters often have depressive tendencies. Alcoholics often suffer from symptoms of low mood, and although alcohol may appear at first as a stimulant and mood enhancer, it is in fact a depressant and substantially decreases the ability of the body to extract nutrients from the food we eat. Dieters tend to eat very few B-complex-containing foods, and they often suffer from depression as well.

According to Dr. Goldwag there are between eight and twelve specific characteristic signs of more severe depression. "Generally these should be present for at least two weeks and represent a change from a previous state: They are reduction in appetite, reduction in sleep ability, fatigue, lack of energy, agitation or retardation in motor activity, loss of interest in usual activities, loss of interest in sex, feelings of worthlessness or guilt, slowed thinking, inability to concentrate to a severe degree, and recurring thoughts of suicide, or suicide attempts."

Everyone from time to time has one or more of these symptoms. But when approximately four or five of these are present for a long period of time, and when this represents a departure from a person's usual personality, the possibility of depression should be considered.

As Dr. Goldwag reminds us, "The first drugs ever used for treating depression were amphetamines. In their time, before they got such a bad reputation, they were considered helpful. In the old days—20, 30, or 40 years ago—amphetamines were used for weight control. They did diminish the appetite, and they also made a person feel good, alert, and more energetic. People who went on diets and took amphetamines felt great.

"Of course, the problem came when you stopped the amphetamines. People would go into a depression. For that reason amphetamines were recognized to be very habit-forming. In order to feel good a person had to keep on taking them. For many people that still seemed okay, at least for a while. For a fair percentage though, the dose became inadequate as the person started feeling like he or she needed more and more of the drug.

This created all kinds of problems with the body's chemistry.

"There are still some medications on the market that act a little bit like the amphetamines, although they are not anywhere near as powerful. These are mild sympathetic nervous system stimulants that are sold over the counter, such as those people use to keep awake when they have to drive. In some instances I'm sure there are people who take them as a way of counteracting depression.

"The next group of drugs to come along were the tricyclic antidepressants. They're called tricyclic because of their chemical structure, which is a triple cycle. There are a whole bunch of them now on the market. The newer group are those that inhibit the enzymes that break down serotonin. They are designed to try to raise the serotonin level in the brain. In that way they counteract depression.

"They are all to varying degrees effective, but they all have side effects. Some of the side effects are severe; some are mild. They usually take days or weeks before they are effective, and in this way they are different than the amphetamines used to be, because those would work in a matter of minutes or hours. Of course, in the long run the present-day antidepressants may be more effective.

"As far as nutritional protocols, the ones I know of that are of practical use are the ones that use high doses of B complex, specifically niacin. Those have been used for some time now. You have to be a little bit careful of niacin because over long periods of time, in high doses, there can be some effects on the liver.

"The doses of niacin that have been used, mostly by Dr. Hoffer, have been in the ranges of 1 to 3 grams a day. That's thousands of milligrams a day, whereas the requirements for avoiding a deficiency are measured in just 10 or 20 mg."

Dr. Robert Atkins distinguishes two types of depression, each with its respective type of therapeutic approach. "Clinically, you can divide depressions into two different categories: the apathetic depression where you just can't get interested in or enjoy anything, and the agitated or anxious depression, where basically you are depressed and nervous. The latter is responsive to increasing serotonin levels and is best treated with tryptophan. Tryptophan is extremely valuable in cases of agitated depression. Apathetic depression is best treated with tyrosine or what we now call acetyltyrosine, and a product called Noraval."

Dr. Doris Rapp, like many other doctors we interviewed, discerned environmental and nutritional causes of depression. "There is no doubt that certain people become sad when they eat certain foods. One youngster became depressed and nearly suicidal when she was on fluoride tablets. Then she was put on imipramine and she could barely walk. All we did was make an allergy extract of the fluoride and we could change her drawings from happy faces to tear-stained faces and she would start to cry. For two years, the fluoride had been causing her trouble, but none of her doctors would believe that a fluoride tablet could cause this problem. Now fluoride isn't necessarily bad for everybody, but it is certainly not a good preparation for certain individuals.

"I see patients who don't have asthma and hay fever during the pollen season, but they become suicidal and depressed every year at the same time when a certain tree pollinates, when the grass pollinates, on moldy days, and when the ragweed pollinates. So if you can see a pattern to your depression, it is worth trying to figure out what might be the reason for that pattern."

Dr. Michael Schachter describes several alternative courses

of treatment with patients suffering from depression. "Many people who are depressed are often deficient in nutrients or thyroid. By giving them these nutrients, their depression frequently is alleviated, sometimes in just one or two visits. Often you don't need to go to drugs, although sometimes you will. Sometimes depression is caused by a deficiency of the neurotransmitter for norepinephrine. In such a case the amino acid L-tyrosine, or the amino acid DL-phenylalanine may be helpful. DL-phenylalanine consists of two forms of phenylalanine, namely D-phenylalanine and L-phenylalanine. L-phenylalanine is used by the body to make proteins. D-phenylalanine is a precursor of the brain substance D-phenylethylamine, which is frequently deficient in people who are suffering from depression. I also recommend the mineral magnesium, and vitamin B_1 (thiamine) for depression. But the course of treatment really has to be individualized.

"You also want to clean up the diet and eliminate sugar, artificial sweeteners and other nonphysiologic chemicals, white flour products, caffeine, and other harmful substances. The overgrowth of the microorganism candida albicans is often an important factor in people who are depressed. Many patients who have candida problems are also depressed. Oral antibiotics, oral contraceptives, and steroids predispose a person to chemical imbalances and an overgrowth of candida, or yeast, which is frequently manifested as abdominal gas and bloating, chronic vaginitis in women, and depression. Frequently I will treat it with an anti-candida diet, eliminating sugar and yeast products and using a variety of anti-candida nutrients. Sometimes I'll use anti-candida medications. This regimen will frequently clear up the depression, as well as many of the other symptoms."

Dr. Lendon Smith addresses some of the more baffling

aspects of depression in today's society. "The more we hear about the rising tide of suicides in adolescents and even in children as young as eight, nine, and ten, it seems astounding that such a thing should overwhelm substantial numbers of children in what is supposed to be the happiest time of life. I evaluate children and adults who are depressed. For some of them there is no apparent reason for their overwhelming sadness. They've got good relationships with other people. Their social organization is intact. They've had a good upbringing. They have a good self-image. They have good school or work performance and they're getting nice accolades from relatives and friends. Why are they depressed? It just doesn't seem right.

"When we do blood tests on these people we find, in general, that there are two things wrong. One is that they're nutrient deficient. In the particular program I'm doing, we go by the deviation from the mean. If, for instance, calcium's range is 8.5 to 10.5, then 9.5 is the mean. If they're down to 9 or 8.6, the doctor will say, 'Everything is okay.' Still, if there are enough of those scores below the mean, these people don't have enough wherewithal, enough nutrients, to satisfy all their enzyme requirements.

"Fifteen years ago, for example, a 20-year-old woman came to see me who was depressed for no apparent reason. She came from a good family, and had a nice boyfriend and a good job. Everything seemed fine but she would still get depressed every once in a while.

"At that time I was experimenting with vitamins. I thought it would be quite safe to give her a shot of the mixed B complex vitamins. I included a cc of everything from B_1 to folic acid and B_{12}. I would give about 50 mg of each one of these vitamins and 50 mcg of the B_{12} intramuscularly every day.

"After two or three of these shots this patient told me that the treatment wasn't working very well for her. She asked, 'Couldn't you give them as separate vitamins?' I started giving her injections of isolated vitamins. I gave her a shot of 100 mg of B_1 on Monday and B_2 on Tuesday. I gave her separate shots of B_3, B_6, B_{12}, and folic acid.

"She reported feeling terrible after receiving B_1, thiamine. She asked me never to do that again. I thought that seemed odd. After the B_2 she came back and said that it was okay but nothing special. She said the same thing after receiving the B_3. But after B_6 she came back and said, 'I think you're onto something.' She also really liked the B_{12} and the folic acid.

"These three vitamins were the important ones for her. I mixed them up and gave them to her every week or two. With that combination, she was apparently satisfied.

"About five or six years ago, I started a new program where we have people smell vitamins to see what they need. If it's a good smell or no smell, they need it. If it's a bad smell, they don't.

"I had her open up thiamine and smell it. She said, 'Good lord. Somebody must have done something awful to this.' I explained to her that nothing was wrong with the vitamin but that she didn't need it. She had some bacteria in her intestinal tract that helped her make her own thiamine. Her body was therefore rejecting it. B_3 had no smell; she needed that. B_6 had a good smell; she needed that. B_{12} and folic acid had no smell so she needed that. Her body told her what she needed, and she could satisfy its requirements. Apparently this method of using the sense of smell and taste is highly accurate in determining people's needs. It should be used rather than just taking multivitamins willy-nilly.

"Craving chocolate is also a sign of depression. It usually

means that people need magnesium, because there's magnesium in chocolate. Women, the day before their menstrual period, often find themselves searching through the cupboards for chocolate. They find a big canister of Hershey's and drink it down before feeling better from the magnesium.

"I often had the delightful experience of giving an intravenous mixture of vitamin C, calcium, magnesium, and B vitamins. Usually it has more magnesium than calcium. Afterwards I asked patients whether they would like some chocolate and they told me they didn't need it. It really is connected.

"Women in the sixth month of pregnancy will often send their husbands out for ice cream because the baby is starting to grow fast. The woman has a conscious need for dairy products because she knows they will bring her the calcium she needs, but she also says, 'Don't forget the pickles.' She knows, somehow, that she needs to acidify that calcium source for the baby. She will not get much out of it and she will suffer from leg cramps.

"The chemist I work with in Spokane discovered something about GGT, a liver and gallbladder enzyme called gamma glutamil transpeptidase. The range that the lab has is anywhere from 0 to 40. They find these values all over the place. The mean would be about 20.

"What we've found is that if their level is below 20, they're more likely to have some of these magnesium deficiency symptoms—short attention span, trouble relaxing or sleeping, little muscle cramps in the feet and legs, and a craving for chocolate. Most of these people don't like to be touched. They may be a little crabby. Those symptoms go with low magnesium.

"Magnesium is one of the first minerals to disappear from food when it's been processed. Magnesium is also one of the first minerals to leave the body when there is stress, which accounts for how many women behave a day or so before their periods. They feel stressed because they're losing their magnesium.

"We need to supply magnesium to these people. We can determine who needs it by the blood test and by the sense of smell. If people smell a bottle of pure magnesium salt— magnesium chloride is a good one—if it smells good or if there's no smell, then the person needs it. The blood test we usually use is the 24 chem. screen, the standard blood test.

"Many symptoms of depression, hyperactivity, headaches, loss of weight, and other conditions are related to genetic tendencies. If there is a tendency to be depressed in the family, a magnesium deficiency will allow that tendency to show up. If there's alcoholism, diabetes, obesity in the family, then low magnesium may allow those things to show up in a person. There are reasons to explain all these things and nutrition is basic to this. The patients don't have an antidepressant pill deficiency; they usually have a magnesium deficiency.

"The first thing I do is ask people what they're eating. If I find that they're eating a lot of dairy products, and that as a child they had their tonsils taken out, and that they had a lot of strep throat and ear infections, then I know they're allergic to milk and they're looking for calcium. Sure enough, the blood tests will show this. That's the first thing they have to stop. Whatever they love is probably causing the trouble because food sensitivities can cause low blood sugar."

Summing up, Dr. Smith cites low blood sugar and magnesium deficiency as two key hidden causes of depression. "As we know—those of us who have worked with nutrition at all—low blood sugar, not just eating sugar, can do that, but also

43

eating foods to which a person is sensitive, will make the blood sugar fall and that can lead to depression. So lack of magnesium and falling blood sugar, for whatever reason, are the two most significant things responsible for a susceptibility to depression."

Depression and Tobacco

Dr. Abram Hoffer tells the story of a classic case of a misdiagnosis corrected, enabling one man to start anew after his previous life had already been ruined. "A high school teacher and principal of about 45 developed a severe depression. In fact, I believe he was misdiagnosed as a schizophrenic. He exhibited what we call a straightforward, deep-seated, endogenous depression. He was in a mental hospital for about a year or two, and then discharged. He was so depressed that no one could live with him. His wife divorced him and eventually he was living with his aunt, who looked after him as if he were a child. As a last resort, he was referred to me.

"When he came to see me, which was many years ago, I had just started looking into the question of allergies. At that time, I wasn't very familiar with food allergies, but I thought he was a very interesting case and I said to myself, 'He is a classic case of a depression, maybe schizophrenic. He'd be the last person in the world who would respond to this anti-allergy approach.' At that time I was using—and I still do—a four-day water fast. This is a way of determining whether or not these allergies are present. He agreed that he would do the fast, which also involved refraining from any smoking or consuming of alcohol; he had to drink about eight glasses of water a day and nothing else. His aunt said she would help make sure he complied. When he came back to see me two weeks later, he and his aunt explained that, at the end of the four-day fast, he was normal. All of the depression was gone.

"This same man then began to get tested for food allergies and he found that not a single food made him sick. But now he began to smoke again. Within a day after he resumed smoking, he was back in his deep depression. The ironic thing was that he had a brother who was a tobacco company executive, who kept sending him free cartons of cigarettes. Now when we made the connection to his cigarette smoking, he stopped smoking. Thirty days later, after he had been depressed for four years and hadn't been able to work, he was back in school teaching. And I remember this clearly because the insurance company that was then paying his monthly pension was so astounded at this dramatic response that they sent one of their agents to see me, to find out what the magic wand was that I had waved to get this patient off their rolls. This is a classic case of an allergy to tobacco that was causing this man's depression."

Effect of Exercise, Nutrition, and Proper Lifestyle on Depression

Dr. William Goldwag insists on the importance of those changes which can be made by the patient himself or herself. "When we have patients who are depressed and we can get them moving, the depression is greatly alleviated. Of course, drugs have changed the whole treatment of depression greatly, but the impact exercise can have on depression has often been overlooked, and it needs to be re-emphasized. People who are on antidepressants may improve, but the way for them to really get back to functioning well—back in touch with their environment, back to work, back in relationships with their family—is to get them moving. And there's no better way to get people moving than through exercise, whose healing potential has no limits.

"The individual is the important thing to take into account when I recommend exercise. There is no one exercise that is good for everybody. Some people can just do a little bit; some can push themselves much further. Ask anybody who has gone from a relatively sedentary life to an exercise program and they will all report the same thing: more energy, more interest in what is going on, a clearer mind, and less stress. Being active, therefore, is an integral part of any kind of medical program, particularly for people who are having mental disturbances.

"I have many patients who have had very stressful medical histories or emotional histories. Today, as more and more people are revealing the difficulties they had as children—the abuse, both sexual and nonsexual—their history, and the stress it causes based on these early childhood experiences continues to have an impact on their lives. Even though their lives may be relatively serene now, psychically they are still dealing with a lot of these issues.

"At the same time, they have to be made to realize that nutrition plays an integral role in their feeling well. They have to supply their bodies with proper nutrients and eliminate excesses or chronic addictions to alcohol, drugs, or food (including sweets and sugar). Inevitably, I find that if someone gets away from an addiction to sugar, they function much better. The old term hypoglycemia is very appropriate for their condition, particularly for people with chronic depression, chronic fatigue syndrome, and chronic immune system dysfunction. These people find that when they modify their diets and get off sugars, their mental functioning improves considerably.

"This is the first step: switching to a healthy diet containing lots of vegetables, fruits, and whole grains, and minimizing the amount of meat in the diet. Now some people will feel better once they modify their diet, and they'll be able to move right into more activity. Some people need to start off with some kind of moderate exercise program and almost automatically they will start to look for a more nutritious diet. The two seem to go hand in hand. Nowadays, so many athletes are paying a lot more attention to what they eat, in addition to their workouts. Similarly, many people who are paying attention to their diets now find that exercise almost becomes an inevitable consequence of paying attention to promoting good health.

"After paying attention to exercise and nutrition, you need to be aware of the stresses of your own lifestyle: your own patterns of behavior and how they are manifested and how they may be altered by more healthy ways of thinking. For example, if you frequently get upset by dwelling on the past, then you need to try not to think so much about what took place in the past or what is going to happen in the future. Your emotional work is to learn how to focus on the present reality, what's going on now, by putting the body in a mode where it is accepting what's happening now, so you're ready for anything that may happen, instead of reliving crises over and over again."

5. *Eating Disorders*

Anorexia and Bulimia

Anorexia nervosa and bulimia are pernicious conditions that are pervasive in our consumption-centered society, affecting women in particular, especially younger women and teenagers. Several physicians practicing orthomolecular psychiatry have approached these conditions in terms of zinc deficiency. Dr. Michael Schachter has stated that "some people who suffer from an eating disorder may be suffering from a zinc deficiency. A few years ago, Alex Schauss presented a paper about a number of patients who were suffering from anorexia nervosa. He found that they were zinc-deficient by using a simple test called a zinc taste test. The person holds a small quantity of zinc sulfate solution in his or her mouth. If the individual describes it as having a bad taste, then he or she usually has adequate levels of zinc in the tissues. On the other hand, if the person can't taste the solution or if it tastes just like water, then he or she may have a zinc deficiency. Even if his or her blood levels look fine, zinc tissue levels may be low. Schauss found he had trouble correcting these zinc abnormalities with zinc tablets or capsules, and needed to use the liquid zinc sulfate solution, which seemed to be absorbed.

"A zinc deficiency often results in a vicious cycle because the zinc deficiency actually inhibits one's ability to absorb zinc in capsule or tablet form. However, the zinc sulfate solution seems to be absorbed, resulting in both clinical improvement and an improved ability to absorb oral zinc tablets or capsules. While I haven't seen many patients in the last couple of years with anorexia nervosa, I have had people with milder loss of appetite, and sometimes excessive appetite, who have had zinc deficiencies. I have been able to rely on this test and administering zinc liquid to improve the condition of these patients," Dr. Schachter concludes.

On the subject of bulimia, Dr. Doris Rapp also discusses the importance of zinc. Zinc deficiency may be a factor, even though the stated reason for the behavior is avoidance of weight gain. According to Dr. Rapp, "In cases where youngsters or adults are eating and then purging themselves in the bathroom by putting a finger down their throats, these individuals are ostensibly getting rid of the food because they don't want to gain weight. But some studies have suggested that zinc can be a helpful form of treatment."

Dr. José Yaryura-Tobias reminds us of the life-threatening severity of a condition like anorexia nervosa, and of his view that any nutritional approach must be preceded by a program of cognitive therapy. "Anorexia nervosa, from our perspective, is an obsessive-compulsive disorder that is related to self-image, the way that we perceive ourselves. Basically, anorexia nervosa is the process by which a human being self-starves. Thirty percent of the population who self-starve eventually die.

"From the biochemical viewpoint, in the vast majority of cases when patients come for a consultation they are already very emaciated. The chemistry we can measure is very altered. We know that there is a groove that is related to an area of the brain called the limbic system. This is the hypothalamic area, which regulates sugar, thirst, appetite, and so forth. This information can help us classify some of these patients, but does not tell us how to manage and eventually cure the problem. The rest of the problem, we feel, has to do with body image perception, the way that these patients see their own bodies. They feel too fat, too slim. They have different perspectives than the rest of us.

"How do we treat this condition? Basically we use a nutritional approach after the patient has undertaken a behavioral program with cognitive therapy. Cognitive therapy is important because the idea is to educate the person about their problems and to discuss with them how many false beliefs they have about who they are, why they think this way, why their body looks the way it does for them, and so forth. So false-belief modification is an important part of treatment."

Food Addiction

As I have said and written for many years, food cravings and food addictions often mask food allergies to the very same foods we crave. (See earlier books of mine, such as *The Complete Guide to Sensible Eating* and *Good Food, Good Mood*.) For the present discussion, I've found holistic practitioners who include in their practice ways of treating food addiction.

One such physician, Dr. Hyla Cass, describes her experience treating patients suffering from food addiction as follows: "Some time ago, a psychologist who specializes in eating disorders began to send her clients to me because she had heard that antidepressant medications worked for these patients. I had shifted to a more holistic way of looking at things, so I told the psychologist that before I did anything with antidepressants I would try some other things. With certain eating disorders, such as food cravings, the underlying problem is a food allergy. *We often crave the very foods to which we are allergic.* Typically, it's the very things we want to eat that are the most damaging, that create the symptoms. In fact, it's like an addiction to alcohol: As you abstain from the foods you're addicted to, you begin to have withdrawal symptoms and crave those foods even more.

"In order to break the cycle in cases of food addiction, just as when breaking the cycle with drinking (alcoholics are actually allergic to alcohol), you need to supply the body with the appropriate nutrients. When we correct the deficiencies and restore body balance, the food cravings and allergy symptoms will often be relieved. Rather than having to rely strictly on 'willpower,' it is possible for individuals to break addictive cycles by achieving metabolic balance, through avoiding the offending foods and supporting the body with a balanced nutritional program of vitamins, minerals, and amino acids. Often, the cravings will then simply go away. It's quite remarkable: With a good vitamin and mineral product, you can often put a stop to the food allergy and its accompanying symptoms.

"I may order a plasma amino acid analysis, a blood test to determine which amino acids—especially among the essential ones which the body cannot synthesize by itself—are low. The amino acid glutamine, in a dosage of 500–1,000 mg, is particularly useful for reducing cravings, including alcohol cravings.

"There are other things to do for food allergies as well," Dr.

Cass adds. "Addictions and allergies are often related to magnesium deficiency and can be corrected by supplementation. There are also techniques that can actually eliminate food allergies through the use of acupuncture and acupressure. As we can see," Dr. Cass concludes, "there are many ways, other than psychotherapy and medication, to approach what at first seems like a psychological problem."

Dr. Doris Rapp brings us more detail concerning the connection between food cravings and allergies: "In my experience, eating disorders and alcoholism can be related to allergies. Frequently, eating disorders are food addictions. When you have a food sensitivity, there is a certain phase of it that makes you really crave that food. And if you happen to be addicted to wheat or baked goods, for example, you can never get enough of them, with the result that you may become obese. To give another example, men who are addicted to corn may drink a lot of beer and they can become alcoholics. They're sensitive to and addicted to the beer, but it's the corn—or sometimes some other component—in the beer that is causing the problem. Sometimes, for those with an allergy to grains, they may feel 'drunk' after eating cereal or certain types of baked goods."

6. Insomnia

Although we spend roughly a third of our lives sleeping, the essential nature of what sleep is still isn't fully understood. Insomnia is a very common symptom of many of the disorders discussed elsewhere in this book, ranging from anxiety to schizophrenia and including various other mood disorders. Typically, anxiety makes it more difficult to go to sleep, and depression can cause early waking. Insomnia can also result directly from physical symptoms such as pain or indigestion, or as a side effect of drug medication.

Dr. Robert Atkins points out the efficacy of tryptophan, which isn't currently legally available in the U.S., in the treatment of insomnia: "Tryptophan is very valuable for sleep disorders because serotonin is the sleep chemical. If you take it right when you are ready to go to bed, when your serotonin level is on the upswing anyway, you are really fitting in physiologically with your body's chemical rhythms."

Most of the doctors I interviewed shared similar experiences in treating insomnia. A major cause of insomnia, especially if it's chronic, is reactive hypoglycemia. This is frequently exacerbated

53

by eating late at night, especially if you eat foods with a high glucose level, such as pastries, candy, or even fruit juice. Such foods cause your blood sugar level to go up and then plummet, a fluctuation that can contribute to insomnia. Also, overindulging late at night in highly fatty foods can cause sleeplessness. That's because foods with a lot of fat take four to five times longer to empty from the stomach and be digested than simple or complex carbohydrates do.

Another big factor in insomnia is intake of stimulants, such as the caffeine in coffee, tea, chocolate, and even colas, which people consume at all hours without much thought as to the stimulant effects. Alcohol, although generally considered a depressant, can have stimulant effects in some oases.

In addition to food and drink, certain medications as well can be culprits in insomnia. Drugs that interfere with the natural sleep cycle include Prozac, the newer drugs related to it, and Xanax.

Exercising in the evening is another possible bane for the insomnia-prone in that it can overstimulate adrenal levels and excite the musculoskeletal system, resulting in difficulty getting to sleep. Likewise, overstimulating the mind by thinking about unresolved conflicts can be a problem when the goal is sleep.

Concerning ways to reach that goal, herbs that are nontoxic and have no contraindications can be a real help to those challenged by insomnia. Unlike sleeping pills, herbs won't leave you in a fog in the morning, or feeling like you haven't really slept. Passionflower is an important relaxant herb popular in much of Europe. Other possibilities include valerian root, a natural calmative used by orthomolecular psychiatrists for people who tend to be anxious, and hops.

Other things to try: foods with naturally occurring

tryptophan in high amounts; calcium citrate and magnesium citrate—1200 mg of each taken any time after dinner; 50 mg of the B complex; and 200 mg of inositol. Also, 200 mcg of chromium in the evening will help stabilize your blood sugar level.

For those with a partner, a gentle neck and head massage for 15 minutes may do the trick in conquering insomnia, and 15 minutes in a warm bath may be helpful as well (no partner required).

Along the lines of positive affirmation, writing in a diary shortly before bedtime can be extraordinarily beneficial. It can be a way of really seeing what you've done that's affirmed your mental, spiritual, and physical health, as well as any deeds you've done that have had positive effects on others. If a person spends some time at the end of each day reflecting on what they've done in the past 24 hours that's been positive, and on plans for the next day, he or she gains a sense of completeness about the day. In a sense, then, diary-writing legitimizes going to bed; it's as if you can now see that you really deserve the good night's sleep you're about to get.

7. Manic Depression (Bipolar Disorder)

Dr. Garry Vickar describes bipolar disease as an illness that has a manic component and a depressed component. If we want to look at mood disorders as a distinct group, which he describes as useful, we're talking about "diseases of unknown etiology characterized by recurrences of disturbed mood."

"If the mood is one of either agitation or elevated mood," Dr. Vickar continues, "one calls that hypomanic or, at the most extreme, manic. Manic individuals are those whose moods are elevated, with, typically, accompanying disorders of energy, both physical and emotional.

"The opposite pole, which is where this term of polarity comes in, is that of depressed mood. Here, there's slowness of thinking, a lowness of mood, a slowness of motor activity. Of course, there are people whose mood disorders consist of simply one pole, that is, they have recurrent depression.

"The primary problem associated with mood disorders is exactly what it says: There is a problem with mood. Along with that come other features: e.g., people who have depressed moods will also very often end up having slowdowns in body functions, such as disturbances in sleep and reduced appetite for food, sex, and pleasurable pursuits. Depressed people often find that food doesn't taste as good as it once did. They lose their ability to enjoy pleasurable activities, whether these are sports, hobbies, or sexual activity.

"With depression there's an overwhelmingly painful, heavy, loss of one's sense of having the ability to function in the world, a sense of one's uselessness. The danger, of course, is that people may become so overwhelmed by their own subjective experience of loss and uselessness that they think their lives are not worth living or they come to believe that others think that their lives are not worth living. In the worst case, someone will lose perspective and think that the world is so terrible that their loved ones shouldn't live. Then you have the specter of the potential of homicidal/suicidal activities.

"There are illnesses that fall under the rubric of mood disorders that don't have a manic component. These are recurrent depressions. Generally, the incidence of mood disorders, especially depressive disorders, is substantially greater, that is, more common, than schizophrenic disorders. Recurrent depressions certainly occur frequently. Depression is a very serious illness and a very insidious one in which people lose their perspective on themselves and their views of where they fit into the world.

"At the opposite pole of the depression is what I consider a hypomanic state. Today it is uncommon to see people whose illness is so out of control that they become truly manic. More often you will see individuals who are manic-depressive becoming excessively elevated in their moods. They become more expansive. They might go on spending sprees and spend money they don't have, or get involved in activities that they truly are not qualified for. They may run up charge cards, or get involved in gambling, financial affairs, extramarital affairs, alcohol, or possibly drug abuse that they would not otherwise be doing. It becomes almost the reverse of the depression spectrum—they need less sleep, they need less food, and everything is very intense. It can become rather horrific because people can become exhausted. They're sleeping two or three hours a day, if that. They may be getting by on a cup of coffee and a soda and cigarettes. At the same time they have this overwhelming sense of omnipotence about themselves and their abilities. So it can be a very, very dangerous period of time."

As Dr. Vickar reminds us, a manic episode may also take forms very different from the euphoria described above: "It can also be a period when, instead of being overly expansive, people become overly suspicious. They become paranoid. The opposite side of persecutory paranoia is grandiosity. Sometimes the grandiose patient grows irritable, angry, and upset at other people who are getting in the way of the wonderful achievements he or she has to offer the world.

"When treating patients suffering from manic-depression, also known as bipolar disorder, we have certain advantages if we accept that the mood disorders are related to possibly disturbed serotonin metabolism. In Canada they have tryptophan; we used to have it here.

"I don't use other amino acids but I certainly use lithium. Now we're discovering that some of the other anti-seizure medications may work in patients with lithium intolerance. Lithium is a naturally occurring substance so I prefer it over the other anti-seizure medications which are, of course, man-made. In fact, lithium is a perfect example of a naturally occurring substance being used by traditional psychiatrists to treat biochemical diseases. Sometimes you use lithium in schizophrenic patients who also have secondary depressions of their moods. You want to be cautious, however.

"If a patient is manic and having psychotic symptoms, I tend to use a formulation similar to that given to psychotic patients. Lithium is certainly added in large part. If the patient's mood is low and he or she is depressed, lithium is sometimes of value, but not always. In addition to traditional antidepressants, I make sure they have enough B complex vitamins.

"Before tryptophan was taken off the market, I used a fair amount of it. There are some people who use phenylalanine or tyrosine, and these substances can be purchased, but it is often difficult for patients to get them. Not every hospital will stock them for you either. Also, sometimes the quality of the product is hard to verify."

Dr. Vickar describes a case history involving manic depression: "I treated a patient who had, for 40 years, exhibited a history that was very clearly that of a manic depressive: He was erratic, impulsive, had marital problems, and was in and out of jobs. His response came when I added lithium to the vitamins, and nothing else. In over 40 years of his marriage, nobody had ever taken a look at the possibility that he had a biochemical abnormality. They just thought he was immature, or impulsive, or perhaps a bit antisocial. I see him once a year, and he takes lithium and vitamins and nothing else. Lithium is a naturally occurring substance that manic-depressives need in higher doses than the rest of us. So here is a case of somebody who, for the better part of a lifetime of illness, hadn't been diagnosed at all."

8. Obsessive-Compulsive Behavior

Obsessive-compulsive disorders affect about six million Americans. This type of condition is characterized by repetitive thinking and the inability to control or put a stop to this thinking process, which Dr. José Yaryura-Tobias describes as "very forceful, practically taking over the mind. It doesn't allow you to think about anything else. Compulsions are urges that are so extremely demanding that they appear to have to be carried out." Some of the main compulsions are double-checking and hand washing. If the compulsion isn't carried out, there is anxiety that will cease or diminish if it is. This illness has been described in medical literature for at least 200 years.

Dr. Yaryura-Tobias tells us some of the peculiar characteristics of obsessive-compulsive behavior: "It usually takes about seven years or so for a patient to come in for a consultation, which tells us that the condition tends to occur gradually, becoming a part of the patient's behavioral system in a very, very slow manner. It occurs with equal frequency in males and females. Fifty percent of obsessive-compulsive patients manifest their sickness during childhood or adolescence. Later on—primarily after the age of 40—it fades away, and it becomes very rare after the age of 50.

"As to why this condition exists at all, we don't have a sure answer to that question. The behavior may result from a learning process that takes hold during childhood. There is a theory that is now slowly being accepted about a biochemical process at work related to changes in neurotransmitters—the chemical substances in the brain that build bridges between neurons in the nervous cells so that they can transmit signals from the outside into our system or, in the reverse direction, have us act to affect the outside world. The key neurotransmitter that is being studied in this regard is serotonin.

"To treat obsessive-compulsive disorders, behavioral therapy, and an amino acid approach, such as the use of L-tryptophan, would be the treatment of choice, along with some other medications.

"We basically treat with behavioral therapy. We try to use thought-stopping, exposure (flooding) and response prevention to prevent the brain from repeating the same thought. That is difficult, so we also use cognitive therapy to explain the reasons we think the things we do, and try to modify the thought.

"Compulsions are the area where behavioral therapy is most effective. We expose the patient, either in reality or in his or her imagination, to face what he is afraid of. If you have fears of AIDS or of blood, you are exposed to blood or taken to the hospital where there might be patients with AIDS. Or you will read articles on the condition.

"If it is contamination from dirt the patient is afraid of, we teach the person how to touch objects and not to be afraid of them. Then we prevent the patient from washing their hands; in other words, they must remain unclean for awhile. I'm talking about patients who, when they are seriously ill, might completely use up one or two bars of soap per day. They might engage in rituals of washing for many hours. They may wash their hands sometimes a hundred or more times a day. Some of these patients, in addition, will clean their hands with alcohol or other substances. Sometimes their skin becomes extremely raw. I've seen cases where patients require plastic surgery.

"Overall, the treatment takes about six months. With medication there is improvement up to 60 or 70 percent of the time.

"My colleagues and I were the first to use tryptophan and with it we were able to reduce and almost eliminate completely the use of drugs for this condition, and we obtained very good results. Unfortunately, tryptophan has been banned so we can no longer use it. We were using between 3000 and 9000 mg per day.

"Then we used vitamin B_6, 100 mg, three times a day. Vitamin B_6, pyridoxine phosphate, is a vitamin that is very important for the breakdown of tryptophan into serotonin. The idea behind this was that either these patients didn't have enough serotonin in their brains, were very dependent on serotonin, or that the normal conversion of tryptophan into serotonin was not occurring.

"When we found by measuring that there was a lack of serotonin, this could be reversed by the administration of L-tryptophan with niacin and vitamin B_6. Some medications also accomplish this result, but with medications we face many types of side effects.

"About 30 percent of patients do not respond to any form of therapy. But it is not a closed chapter for these patients either. An investigation has to be conducted. Now that we have brain imaging, we are able to visualize the brain. We can measure, for instance, the metabolism of sugar in the brain. We find, for instance, the frontal and temporal lobes and the basal ganglia, that are related to Parkinson's disease, disrupted. We see the metabolism of the breakdown of sugar and also images of an abnormal brain. The same can be seen with some electrophysiological measurements of brain wave tests and so forth.

"Interestingly," Dr. Yaryura-Tobias concludes, "work has been going on using pure behavioral therapy before and after measuring serotonin. With just behavioral therapy, we were able to modify the levels of serotonin in the body. In other words, we may not need medication to change or challenge the presence of a neurotransmitter such as serotonin. Simply the mere interaction of behavioral technique may have an effect."

According to Dr. Robert Atkins, there is some common ground between conventional Western medicine and more holistic approaches such as orthomolecular psychiatry, or what he refers to as "complementary" medicine. "Both orthodox medicine and complementary medicine, which is the nutrition-based alternative to orthodox medicine, recognize that if a certain neurotransmitter is in short supply, certain syndromes will result. A classic example is that the serotonin-deficient person will often be an obsessive-compulsive. These are the people who can't get out of the house because they've got to make sure the light switches are off or the gas jet isn't on—the people who have to wash their hands 20 times a day, and whose desks have to be perfectly neat. These same people are serotonin-deficient."

The difference between the conventional and the alternative medical communities lies in how they address the problem. Dr. Atkins describes the conventional approach: "Now there are drugs that block the degradation of serotonin and allow the serotonin level to lift, but these drugs do a lot of other things: They poison a lot of enzyme systems and that's why so many people got into trouble with Prozac and drugs like that." And the more enlightened alternative approach: "However, you can increase serotonin with the nutrition precursor, tryptophan, which, unfortunately, the FDA took off the market because of a bad batch.

"Dr. Russell Jaffe has done research to indicate that the best treatment for the bad tryptophan syndrome (the easinophilia myalgic syndrome) is the use of pure unadulterated tryptophan. People with obsessive-compulsive and anxiety disorders often improve on tryptophan. Since the FDA ban on tryptophan, pure tryptophan has not been available in the United States, even by prescription. However, some pharmacies will compound capsules of 5-hydroxy tryptophan. This compound is an intermediary between tryptophan and 5-hydroxy-tryptamine, which is serotonin, the neurotransmitter you are trying to build up. The whole idea of supplying a precursor to build up a neurotransmitter that is in short supply is a fruitful approach to treating psychiatric disorders and should, in my opinion," concludes Dr. Atkins, "be considered before the use of nonphysiologic psychotropic drugs, which have more potential for toxicity."

9. Schizophrenia

Schizophrenia is a group of illnesses of unknown cause that have as their common features disorders of perception and emotion. Schizophrenic illnesses are classified, according to common terminology, as paranoid or nonparanoid, and they are termed either chronic or acute. According to Dr. Garry Vickar, "The new research that's being done suggests that there are, in fact, differences in prognosis" —in other words the likely outcome for patients suffering from schizophrenia— "in part related to the shape of the brain itself, the age at onset, and complicating factors relating to any co-existing drug abuse or other concurrent conditions.

"Clearly," Dr. Vickar continues, "schizophrenic illnesses as a group are among the most serious biochemical disorders there are; it can be said that schizophrenia is to psychiatry what cancers are to general medicine. The bulk of the lost revenue to society, the bulk of psychiatric expense, and the sheer horror to the families, which is not easily quantifiable, are unfortunately all consequences associated with the diagnosis of schizophrenia.

"The most disturbing part of schizophrenia is the

disturbance of thought. These are patients who may have vague symptoms, who go through periods of what German psychiatrists used to call 'stage fright,' and then something happens and they start to believe that their disordered perceptions represent true events. Their strong belief in these disordered perceptions transforms them into delusions, which are simply fixed, false beliefs. Patients will start to believe their delusions and then start to believe their misinterpretation of a perceptual nature. They may hear a voice and believe that the voice is real and represents some real event or real person. They'll act on that. An example would be, if I hear somebody calling my name, if I don't think it's my thought anymore but that there really is somebody calling my name, I will act accordingly. If I think that people are looking at me and making faces, I might think there is something very wrong with me and feel bad or upset about it. If I'm eating my meal and there's a piece of moldy cheese, I might think I've been poisoned and that someone did it to me purposefully. The process starts to escalate and snowball.

"The most diabolical part of the illness is the loss of insight, loss of the ability to reality-test. For instance, if you're driving down the street at night and it's dark and hard to see, and you see something at the side of the road, you might slow down to be cautious, thinking that somebody is going to cross the street. Then you get close enough and see that it's really just shrubs or a mailbox or just part of the normal landscape, and you say, I'm glad I was cautious. If instead, however, you start to distort the original perception and really believe that there's someone who might jump out on the road or that somebody is trying to hurt you and can get in the way of your vehicle, you might take evasive action. In the process, you could have an accident or cause somebody else to have one. You start to distort things without realizing that you are distorting them. That's similar to what happens when the really disastrous part of the illness takes over.

"When you become paranoid and don't know why, you begin to wonder, 'What is it about me that's so bad? Why are people saying bad things about me?' It can become very serious. I had a patient who believed that then-President Reagan was making comments about him—about this individual—and he felt compelled to call the White House and protest to the FBI that he was being hounded by President Reagan. He firmly believed it. When he recovered he didn't believe it, but when he was delusional be firmly believed that the President was, in fact, personally interfering with his life. Such paranoid delusions can become all-consuming and unfortunately very painful."

Dr. Philip Hodes sketches the history of the treatment of schizophrenia in orthomolecular psychiatry as follows: "In the field of schizophrenia, in the 1950s there were three pioneers in orthomolecular psychiatry: Dr. Abram Hoffer, Dr. Humphry Osmond, and Dr. John Smythies, who used large amounts of niacinamide, vitamin C, and some of the other B vitamins, to help their schizophrenic patients recover. In the 1970s, Dr. Alan Cott went to Russia and brought back the practice of fasting, and helped to detoxify many of the brains of schizophrenics who had not responded to any other kind of treatment. He helped them clear their brains so that they became rational and normal.

"Today we live in a state of environmental pollution. There are over 90,000 chemicals in the external environment that we ingest through what we eat, drink, and breathe. Contaminants are in the soil, water, air, and food supply. The particles which are toxic penetrate and leak through the blood brain barrier over time and get into the brain. This process also happens with several of the heavy toxic metals, such as lead, cadmium, copper, iron, arsenic, mercury, and aluminum. These chemicals and heavy metals, by affecting brain chemistry, affect the mind and behavior, so they must be removed. They need to be chelated out.

"In the Science Section of *The New York Times*, on April 27, 1993, an article stated, 'New suspect in bacterial resistance, amalgam. The mercury in dental fillings may spur resistance to antibiotics.' Dr. Hal Huggins has shown that the silver mercury dental amalgams are very harmful; when you chew, the mercury is released, causing immune suppression and brain poisoning. Many of the people who have developed so-called 'mental illnesses' are suffering from things like mercury, lead, copper, iron, and aluminum poisonings. These toxic metals affect one's thinking and behavior. People can develop bizarre behavior and distorted thinking, along with warped perceptions, as a result of these toxic metals. Add to this toxic stew all the insecticides, pesticides, and herbicides that we ingest daily.

"The orthomolecular approach to schizophrenics is to detoxify them, change their diets, and remove foods that are chemically treated, or that contain a lot of sugar and refined carbohydrates, or that have been laced with pesticides. Then these patients are placed on the optimal doses of nutrients for their individual bodies. The nutrients used include vitamin B complex—especially thiamine, niacin, pyridoxine (B_6), and B_{12}.

"The late Dr. Henry (Hank) Newbold demonstrated that many of his schizophrenic psychiatric patients were suffering from a vitamin B_{12} 'dependency' and that they needed large amounts in order to feel well and sane again. Then as the years went by, orthomolecular doctors discovered that the essential minerals—macro minerals such as calcium and magnesium, as well as the trace mineral elements zinc, manganese, chromium, and selenium—also helped balance the cerebral chemistry of schizophrenics. Dr. Priscilla Slagle published her research in a book, *Up From Depression*, showing the important role of amino acids in the brain, and in the treatment of manic depressives and schizophrenics.

"You also have to look at the water supply. Many water supplies contain chemicals, such as iron, silicone, aluminum, fluoride, and chlorine. We ingest all of these things and once they hit the blood stream, they are rushed to all of the 64 to 67 trillion cells in the body. These toxins block out the opportunity for the vital nutrients to be absorbed.

"The basic constituents of the human body are proteins, amino acids (the building blocks of proteins), carbohydrates, fats, vitamins, minerals, oxygen, enzymes, nucleic acids, water, and electromagnetic and biomagnetic energy forms. If any of these are unbalanced or deficient, and there are nutritional deficiencies, different conditions and diseases can arise. Our diet is not really a healthy diet: the soil our food is grown in has been overworked; there have been artificial fertilizers put in; and the foods are refined, processed, and sprayed with all kinds of chemicals and inundated with all kinds of food coloring and dyes.

"When we eat these foods we become both malnourished and toxic. In answer to those who say, 'Oh, you don't need vitamins. Just eat a well-balanced diet,' I say you can't get a well-balanced diet and you do need extra nutrients to help stave off the deleterious effects of all the chemical pollutants in the environment. With orthomolecular therapy," Dr. Hodes concludes, "many people feel a lot better when they get more nutrients than their diet gives them."

Dr. Abram Hoffer reminds us that very early treatment efforts involving orthomolecular psychiatry existed and were critical to the field's current resurgence: "The orthomolecular treatment of schizophrenia was started in Saskatchewan in 1951 when we ran the first double-blind controlled experiments in North American medicine and also the first in worldwide psychiatry. On the basis of these experiments, where we compared the effect of vitamin B_3 against a placebo, we found that the addition of the vitamin to the standard treatment of that day, which was only electroconvulsant therapy, doubled the two-year recovery rate from 35 percent to 70 percent. That was the beginning.

"After that we ran another three double-blind controlled experiments. Since that time we have accumulated massive clinical experience; I myself have seen many thousands of schizophrenic patients. The treatment for the schizophrenic patient is really relatively simple. It's a combination of the best of modern psychiatry, which includes the proper use of tranquilizers, antidepressants, or other drugs, with proper attention to diet and the use of nutrients.

"The main nutrient is vitamin B_3, which has to be given in large quantities. It's not enough to give the tiny amount present in food. One will have to give many thousands of times as much in the standard dose. For the patients I work with, I give 3000 mg per day of either nicotinic acid or nicotinamide, which are both forms of vitamin B_3.

"I also use vitamin C at the same dose level and sometimes a lot more because vitamin C is a very good water-soluble antioxidant. It is considered the foremost, the most active water-soluble antioxidant present in the human body. That's extremely important.

"In many cases," Dr. Hoffer continues, "we use vitamin B_6 as well for a particular group of schizophrenic patients. This is combined with an overall nutritional approach that may also include the use of a very important mineral, zinc. Zinc and B_6 function together and are extremely important.

"Finally, we use manganese to protect our patients against developing tardive dyskinesia. This is a condition which afflicts chronic schizophrenic patients who are placed upon large quantities of tranquilizers. According to Dr. Richard Kunin from San Francisco, when you take tranquilizers for a long period of time you take manganese out of the body, which is the reason patients develop tardive dyskinesia. When you give them back the manganese this condition goes away in most cases.

"I put my patients on a diet that is junk-free. I exclude any of the prepared foods that contain additives, including sugar. I also pay attention to patients' allergies, because 50 or 60 percent of all schizophrenics have major food allergies. If these are not detected and eliminated, the patients are not going to get any better.

"This is essentially the treatment for schizophrenia, although there is one more important variable—the patients themselves. You have to take a lot of time dealing with schizophrenic patients. I will just briefly review what I have done recently. I have re-examined 27 of my chronic schizophrenic patients who have been working with me for at least ten years. They had been sick an average of seven years before they came to see me. They had all failed to respond to any of the standard treatments—drugs, tranquilizers, or shock treatments. They had not been given any vitamins.

"I did a survey of what happened to them after being with me for ten years. Of the 27 really chronic patients, 17 today are normal. They really are well. They're paying taxes. As an example, one man from eastern Canada was a very paranoid schizophrenic. He was in and out of the Ontario mental hospital system. He was so sick that his wife divorced him and his family disowned him. He moved out west to Victoria and was living as a homeless person there for awhile.

"He came under my care and remained on the vitamins, to my surprise. Three or four years ago he got his degree at the local university here and the last time I saw him he was looking for a job. I think this is quite an accomplishment for someone who was a very sick patient.

"Another patient was a woman who, in a psychotic frenzy, burned down her house. She now runs her own business and supervises 12 people. These are examples of some of the recoveries we've had.

"The other ten are not well yet. Some may never be well because they've been sick for too long, but they're certainly an awful lot better than they were when we found them. They're now comfortable. They're able to live with any hallucinations or delusions they still have.

"This is a very chronic group of patients, the kind that normally don't respond. The important thing—going back to the view that you have to expect slow, progressive improvement rather than any sudden cure—is that it took five to seven years of continuous treatment before they reached their current stage of improvement.

"Acute patients, patients who have only been sick for a year, do a lot better, of course," Dr. Hoffer reminds us. "I fully expect that if I see 100 schizophrenic patients who have been sick a year or two or less, after two years of this kind of treatment, 95 percent of them will be well. In fact, the 17 young men and women I mentioned above who made complete recoveries had all become schizophrenic in their teens. They were placed upon vitamin treatment in various parts of Canada and the United

States. These 17 young men and women all went into medicine. Today they are practicing psychiatry. One went to Harvard Medical School and is now a doctor in Boston. One became a president of a major psychiatric association in North America. The other members of that association did not know that he had a history of having been psychotic at one time. That's a pretty good record."

Dr. Garry Vickar emphasizes the holistic foundation of the treatment approach he prefers. "I think in any chronic illness, such as schizophrenia, you have to maximize the person's whole functioning. You want to make them as healthy as possible. You don't want to have an imbalance where your left arm is really maximally in shape because you're a pitcher but the rest of you is flab. You have to have the whole organism as healthy as possible.

"If, in fact, people have abnormal thinking because of deficiencies of B_{12}, maybe they have a lack of an enzyme in their stomach that doesn't carry out the necessary conversion of B_{12} into what the body needs. These people have a disease called pernicious anemia that can result in their becoming paranoid. Once in awhile you'll find a person who lacks this thing called intrinsic factor. You have to give B_{12} supplements to prevent them from becoming paranoid and from developing nervous system signs and symptoms and gait disturbances. With B_{12} they get better. So there are simple things like that which can be done and which, in this modern age, can get overlooked by conventional physicians.

"I check for magnesium levels in all my patients, especially adolescents who drink a lot of soda pop. I also do zinc, copper, and manganese levels because there is some evidence that low manganese is implicated in tardive dyskinesia. A low magnesium level is implicated in irritability, nervousness, even nerve conduction problems and seizures. The worst-case scenario is a premenopausal woman who just had a baby, was on birth control pills prior to her pregnancy, is on prenatal vitamins, and goes back on the pill after the baby is born. She'll have sky-high copper levels, almost toxic relative to zinc.

"With the schizophrenic patient I use niacinamide or niacin (more frequently niacinamide because most patients won't tolerate niacin). I tend to use much of what Abram Hoffer has come up with. I look for a minimum of 3000 mg of niacinamide a day with an equal amount of vitamin C. I recommend a B complex with 50 to 150 mg of the entire B complex, mineral balance, depending upon zinc and copper levels. We try to titrate a dose until we reach a level of improvement with the least amount of medicine and the amount of vitamin and mineral supplements that the patient can tolerate."

Dr. Vickar continues, expressing the broad philosophy of his treatment of schizophrenic patients: "I have patients who have been diagnosed as having schizophrenia, and while I don't argue with the diagnosis, it hasn't captured the whole essence of what is going on with that patient. I prefer to see it as an incomplete diagnosis, rather than as a misdiagnosis. Very often the goal, in the schizophrenic diagnosis, is just to subdue behavior. When people are in such states of distress that their behavior is inappropriate, or agitated, or out of control, the goal is primarily to treat that behavior. I think that there is more we can do. We have to try to understand why the patient is doing what he or she is doing—not necessarily psychologically, but in some way biochemically.

"We don't know what the ultimate causes of schizophrenia are. Each new drug that comes along throws the current theory into such disarray that it doesn't apply anymore, because the new drug doesn't work the way that those preceding it did. So I don't think that anybody knows the causes, but there is one thing that we are sure of: We can make a big difference in how a schizophrenic is doing by applying two basic principles, as Dr. Hoffer has indicated: good sound nutrition and vitamin supplements.

"These are not synonymous. Nutrition has to be the floor upon which the treatment is built. Then, after that, you have to start looking at other factors—whether it be smoking, co-existing alcohol-related problems, dietary disturbances, or absorption difficulties. Also, the patient may not be doing well because what they have been given is, in fact, creating more problems. So we have to be sensitive to such reactions to treatment and continue to modify the treatment all the way along. And again, the approach I find to be most useful is that schizophrenia is not so much a missed diagnosis as it is an incomplete one."

Schizophrenia and Alcoholism

Dr. Abram Hoffer estimates that about ten percent of all schizophrenic patients are also alcoholic. "It's not a big figure," he adds, "if you remember that ten percent of all adults in North America are probably alcoholic. In other words, the same proportion is present in schizophrenics. If you start the other way, a certain percentage of alcoholics are, in fact, also schizophrenic. There is an overlap.

"It has been acknowledged for many years that this particular group that have both problems is very tough to treat. The first person to really show that you can help them was Dr. David Hawkins, who was then practicing on Long Island. He found that when he placed his alcoholic schizophrenic patients on the proper vitamin treatment, including mostly niacin and vitamin C, he began to see a fantastic number of recoveries.

"I have seen some recoveries, but not as many as he has. I can attest to the fact that patients do a lot better if they are treated for both conditions. This treatment includes niacin or niacinic acid and the other vitamins that I use for the treatment of these conditions.

"I think that whether or not they are alcoholic they have to be treated the same way. If they're alcoholic it's vital that they stop drinking. The best way to achieve that is to try to get them to join Alcoholics Anonymous."

"Howard:" A Personal Account of Schizophrenia

"My illness started around 1977, when I developed a persecution complex and delusions of grandeur. I was seeing about three different psychiatrists and they were unable to help me. One psychiatrist thought I was manic-depressive. I wasn't being treated for schizophrenia, which is what I have.

"Dr. Vickar, with the orthomolecular approach, made me well again, and I really owe him a lot. Now I am on a regimen of vitamins and antipsychotic drugs. The vitamins, I am told, enhance the good effects of the drugs so that I don't have to take high doses of the drugs in order to remain normal or stable. Before I got on this regimen I had not been taking any vitamins. Using the orthomolecular approach to help treat my schizophrenia, I basically feel normal and have my life back again."

10. Tardive Dyskinesia

Tardive dyskinesia is a neurological condition which, as its name implies, is one of late onset, that is, tardive. Dyskinesia refers to abnormal movement. Tardive dyskinesia refers to the abnormal neurological movements that occur after a patient has spent a period of time on certain kinds of medicines. When the medicine is reduced or eliminated, the patient starts to demonstrate these abnormal movements. The movements typically involve disturbances around the mouth, the face—involuntary blinking, smacking of lips, twitching around the face. They can occur at varying levels of severity and may involve the entire body.

According to Dr. Garry Vickar, "It used to be said that tardive dyskinesia was untreatable, but that certainly is not true now. Around 15 years ago there was a massive report that showed those physicians in orthomolecular psychiatry who were using vitamins did not have any patients with tardive dyskinesia. We tried to analyze what the factor was that prevented the emergence of TD. At one point, most of us thought that the addition of B_6 might be the factor. Subsequent research has shown that it is probably vitamin E with its antioxidant capacity.

"The patients I've seen with tardive dyskinesia usually come to me after having been treated with drugs for a very long time. These are patients who have been on antipsychotic medications. If they're on an antipsychotic drug and they don't in fact have a psychotic or a schizophrenic illness, they're at higher risk. For example, somebody with a mood disorder given an antipsychotic drug is at higher risk for developing tardive dyskinesia.

"Typically those with tardive dyskinesia are patients who have been treated for schizophrenia over the course of many years. The ravages of the illness are combined with the cumulative effects of the medicine. The older antipsychotic drugs— Thorazine, chlorpromazine, Stelazine, Prolixin, Haldol—work in a certain part of the brain where the neurotransmitter function is tied in with movements. The implication is that treatment with these drugs over the long term can lead to movement disorders.

"Attempts to remedy this have resulted in the creation of newer antipsychotic medications such as Clozaril and Risperdal. These are allegedly less likely to cause tardive dyskinesia because they work on different centers of the brain. They relieve some of the schizophrenic symptoms without the potential for tardive dyskinesia. These drugs haven't been out long enough to know if they will cause other side effects. Clearly we haven't had enough time to know if the newer drugs ultimately will or will not cause similar problems.

"To treat tardive dyskinesia you have to walk a fine line. You have to help patients reinstitute the very medicine that is implicated in causing it to relieve the dyskinesia. Sometimes I call neurologists in. They may have to use, in very interesting combinations, some of the antiseizure medicines that have antispasmodic effects.

"We used to think, many years ago, that the crucial missing

ingredient in patients with tardive dyskinesia was vitamin B_6. It turns out that it is probably vitamin E that is the protective element necessary with regard to TD.

"I treat TD patients with choline and lecithin and large doses of vitamins. The choline and lecithin are tied in with the presumptive mechanism of action of this abnormal movement. If there's an imbalance in the different neurochemical pathways, then it is thought that the choline and lecithin will help along what is called the phosphytotyl choline pathway. You add the lecithin so you don't have to give as much choline, because choline tends to lead to a very fishy smell in the body. It is presumed that this brings a balance back, or re-establishes the proper chemical balance in the brain to relieve the abnormal movements.

"If the chemical pathways in the brain were altered by the use of Haldol and other drugs, there may have been a disturbance of the intricate balance of neurochemicals necessary to coordinate smooth movements. The presumption is that choline and lecithin will help correct the imbalance that was created by the traditional antipsychotic drugs.

"In sum, I use a balance of B vitamins, lots of choline and lecithin, manganese where appropriate, and sometimes I have to call in a neurologist to see what treatments they might want to give, depending on the level of severity of the problem."

ORGANIC CONDITIONS COMMONLY MISDIAGNOSED AS MENTAL DISEASE

11. Blood Sugar Instability (Hypoglycemia)

According to Dr. Hyla Cass, people with hypoglycemia are often diagnosed as though they have simple depression and anxiety, and then treated for a psychological condition. "They are put on anti-anxiety agents such as Valium or Xanax. If they are extremely depressed as well as anxious, they are put on antidepressants such as Prozac. I've had people come to me on medication that wanted to go off of it. It turned out that they were hypoglycemic.

"You can replace antidepressants with amino acids, minerals, and cofactors, vitamins for amino acid metabolism," Dr. Cass adds. "When depressed patients come to see me who are also hypoglycemic, I put them on a hypoglycemic diet, which is approximately six small meals a day. Also, I have them take chromium for balancing their blood sugar levels. I also give them magnesium, glutamine, and tyrosine. Tyrosine is an excellent natural antidepressant. It's a precursor to the neurotransmitter norepinephrine, which is one of the brain chemicals that helps us feel good.

"Hypoglycemia can result from a combination of stress and poor eating habits, particularly in people genetically predisposed to this condition. The disorder can present itself in a variety of ways: depression, irritability, anxiety, panic attacks, fatigue, 'brain fog,' headaches including migraines, insomnia, muscular weakness, and tremors, all of which may be relieved by food. There can be cravings for sweets, coffee, alcohol, or drugs.

"In fact," Dr. Cass continues, "many addictions are related to hypoglycemia. Coffee and sugar consumed by recovering alcohol or drug addicts only prolong their problem, though in a less dangerous, more socially acceptable form. (It is interesting to note the large amount of these substances consumed at Alcoholics Anonymous meetings, for example, and on psychiatric wards.)

"Such individuals can often overcome coffee, drug, and alcohol addiction through correcting their hypoglycemia, *with minimal withdrawal symptoms or later cravings*. For recovering alcoholics, for example, I recommend the hypoglycemic regimen described below plus the amino acid glutamine, 500 mg, three to six times daily, which is particularly useful to counteract cravings.

"The following hypoglycemia program is designed to both strengthen the adrenals and maintain adequate blood sugar levels:

* Elimination of refined carbohydrates (sugar, white flour), coffee, and alcohol.
* Small, frequent meals of complex carbohydrates, high fiber foods, and protein.
* Daily supplementation with a multivitamin/mineral complex that includes (otherwise add) 200–600 mcg chromium, 200–400 mg magnesium, 10–20 mg manganese, 500–1,000 mg potassium, 50–75 mg B

vitamins, 500 mg pantothenic acid (vitamin B$_5$), 3,000
mg vitamin C. These supplements can be divided
into doses taken two to three times daily."

Dr. Leander Ellis suggests that hypoglycemia can be
brought on by a variety of causal factors, some circumstantial,
others stress-related, still others environmental. "Hypoglycemia,"
Dr. Ellis explains, "is a phenomenon that can be triggered by
allergy, infection, exhaustion, or large amounts of sugar that
encourage the growth of yeast in the intestinal tract, which then,
in turn, gives rise to some allergic effects and a variety of other
subtle effects. I see hypoglycemia as a symptom of a larger
problem, rather than as a disease. Most of the time there are
other important causes to account for the roller-coastering of
the blood-sugar levels. The most common one is probably
candida, yeast. The next most likely cause is food allergy. Often,
a person is not only gorging on sugar, but is allergic to sugar, is
not only gorging on chocolate, but is allergic to chocolate. So
you get a curious combination of candida, yeast mold, fungus
allergy, and allergy to foods. You usually have to control these
several elements, as well as to get adequate nutritional support,
in order to quiet these symptoms down.

"Candida is a major factor in hypoglycemia, depression, and
chronic fatigue that the medical profession has continued to
ignore, despite the research results that are available to the
medical community. The major reason for this is that medicine
is taught by prestige suggestion, meaning a doctor needs someone
he or she trusts to tell him what is important. Unfortunately, the
people that we doctors have the most contact with after we leave
medical school are drug company representatives. Therefore,
until a learned professor at an Ivy League medical school tells us
that candida is a problem, it doesn't exist."

Dr. Warren Levin explains the basic physiology of hypoglycemia, as well as some of its special characteristics. "Hypoglycemia is a basic problem that is frequently stress-induced. When people take a large dose of sugar into the body (and one cola drink contains more sugar than the entire bloodstream), the level of sugar in the body goes way up. Now, the body's entire commitment is to maintain balance or equilibrium (the technical word is homeostasis). The body produces a basic hormone called insulin that is supposed to take the sugar from the blood and deliver it into the cells, and when the sugar goes up very rapidly the body reacts excessively, resulting in too much sugar being driven out of the blood, and that produces low blood sugar, or hypoglycemia. The body then has to correct the balance again, and it can be an emergency. If the blood sugar goes too high, it is not an emergency; the body can tolerate it. But the brain requires a certain level of blood sugar to function, so when the blood sugar starts plummeting—and it can sometimes drop at a frightening rate—the body calls forth its emergency hormone, adrenaline.

"Adrenaline was designed to protect us against the saber-toothed tigers back in the primitive world. It mobilizes all sorts of bodily functions. One of the things it does is to dump sugar from the liver into the blood very rapidly. However, adrenaline also causes what we call the fight-or-flight reaction, associated with the state of fear. We get a rapid heartbeat, dry mouth, sweating, fear, and a sense of impending doom."

Dr. Levin then concludes with a cautionary tale that contains precisely the kind of great wisdom and knowledge that the medical community needs to hear: "Now, suppose someone has an ice cream sundae and a few hours later he or she sits down to read the funny papers and all of a sudden he or she gets this terrible reaction. The individual goes to the doctor and explains that while just sitting there, reading the paper, all of a sudden the skin got sweaty and the heart started pounding. The doctor says that the problem is all in the head and that the patient must have a Prozac deficiency. 'With this Prozac prescription,' the doctor adds, 'you'll be fine.' We have to stop thinking that way. Headaches are not a Darvon deficiency, depression is not a deficiency of Elavil, and until doctors realize that the body's biochemistry is an exquisite balancing act, and start treating it with great respect, we are in a lot of trouble. Hypoglycemia is not a disease; it is a symptom requiring a search for an underlying cause."

"William." A Personal Account of Hypoglycemia

"I had been seeing a psychiatrist for depression and was on medication—and still am. I noticed that while the medicine took care of certain symptoms, it seemed to have no effect on an enormous number of them. I used to be a body-builder back in the early 1980s, so I had some experience with nutrition. I went to see Dr. Spreen because I noticed that my hypoglycemia was acting up; I noticed a direct correlation between what I ate and how I felt. When I went to see him, I was complaining of really severe panic disorders, irritability, and difficulty in concentrating. I went from having an excellent memory to no memory at all. Also I had such fatigue it felt like I was walking in Jell-O all the time. I'd sleep 12 hours a day and get up with no energy at all after sleeping. I'd be tired the whole day.

"The first thing Dr. Spreen did was to give me

injections of B$_{12}$. Immediately I noticed a difference. As soon as I'd walk into the gym to work out, my energy was there. In the morning I felt really good. But I was still plagued sometimes by panic attacks. So he put me on a high dose of tyrosine, which is one of the free-form amino acids. I took up to seven grams a day and noticed a real strong response. Tyrosine is also related to the thyroid because one of the products the thyroid needs for normal functioning is tyrosine. He also put me on a low dosage of thyroid, a quarter grain a day. I took that and noticed immediate results. With that and the tyrosine, I felt like a new person.

"This experience showed me that even though a doctor may be treating you for depression, he might be missing the things that might have lead to the depression or that might go hand in hand with it. Many books that I've read—in particular, Carlton Frederick's New Low Blood Sugar and You—*say that when there is any mental disorder present, hypoglycemia is going to be right there along with it. But the medical community doesn't accept that hypoglycemia is as predominant as some nutritionists say it is because the doctors are thinking about the organic forms, which are much rarer. But with the diet that we are eating today, which is high in carbohydrates and low in basically everything good for you, hypoglycemia is manifesting itself in great numbers.*

"As a child, I ate a diet that was full of simple carbohydrates—all sorts of sweets and sugars—and had a lot of the symptoms that are associated with hypoglycemia: I was hyperactive and had asthma.

*You see, hypoglycemia can trigger asthma attacks.
Since I started working out and watching my diet,
the asthma went away.*

*"For the panic attacks, Dr. Spreen suggested
vitamin C. I took vitamin C powder, which is ascorbic
acid, in the morning. I probably took 15 to 20 grams
a day. It was almost like taking a sedative. It calmed
me right down. My thought patterns straightened
out; I was calm; and I wasn't as irritable and fidgety
as I had been. I balanced out the rest of my nutrients
with a mineral supplement and a good vitamin
supplement high in the B spectrum. I take an
additional B complex with pantothenic acid on the
side because Dr. Spreen thinks that most people don't
have enough B vitamins in the diet. I'm inclined to
agree with him, since I've followed his advice and
noticed an enormous positive response."*

12. Candidiasis

Dr. Aubrey Worrell approaches the candida problem holistically: "The body is the source of the candida allergen. We normally live with candida, which inhabits the skin and gastrointestinal tract. A problem arises when there is an imbalance of the candida caused by an overgrowth. When there is more candida than there should be in the gastrointestinal tract, the body absorbs more of the candida antigen. You accelerate the problem by eating sugar and adding foods with mold and by breathing mold in.

"Over a period of years," Dr. Worrell continues, "I noticed that patients with candida manifest multiple symptoms. As an allergist, I would of course see patients with asthma, hay fever, and skin rashes. But I began noticing that many of these patients with allergies had other problems such as respiratory and gastrointestinal symptoms. Another complaint I see quite frequently is people just not feeling good. They're tense or headachy. They're tired and weak. They have a tendency towards depression and fatigue. They're forgetful and unable to concentrate.

"In actuality, these problems are often manifestations of a subtle disruption of immune function in which there's an overgrowth of yeast and an increasing allergy to the mold.

"I place patients with multiple symptoms on a mold-free and yeast-free diet that eliminates foods such as milk and dairy products, particularly cheese. Milk and dairy products are contaminated with mold, and mold is used in the process of cheese-making. I also eliminate yeast breads and yeast foods, as well as vinegars, since these contain a lot of mold allergens.

"If a person is eating a lot of sugar, if he or she has taken a lot of antibiotics, if he or she is not eating a good diet—then the candida is more apt to grow. And that person is likely to have more candida antigen released into their system.

"You have to use a combination of approaches in treating patients with candida. Number one, you have to have a good, nutritious diet. It can't be loaded with alcohol and sugar. It has to be composed of broad-spectrum healthy foods. Number two, you put them on the mold-free diet. Number three, you have to place them on Nystatin therapy for approximately two to six weeks."

Dr. Richard Tan confirms many of Dr. Worrell's insights. Dr. Tan also emphasizes a systemic and holistic approach: "I have been diagnosing a large number of patients with candida, and sugar affects them greatly. Quite a few patients that I am seeing have memory lapses, are forgetful and depressed, and they have seen other doctors who diagnose the depression and give them antidepressants. When I go over all the system reviews, I find that it is more of a systemic problem; along with the candida, they also have some sinus problems, achy bones and joints, stomach upsets, and gas. They often say that they have cravings for sugar or foods that contain sugar, as well as bread.

"I have a survey form that I go through. In my scoring system, after awhile, if the score is high, then I strongly suspect that they have candida. So then I explain my hypothesis and start to treat them. I put them on a diet program plus some anti-fungal medication. When they come back after two weeks, they usually say that they haven't felt so well in a number of years.

"This quick recovery is a revelation to me. I keep on seeing this type of patient. And every time I treat one, I am still amazed at how different they become after awhile, at how much they improve.

"It is estimated that about one-third of the population has candida. I would say that among my patients about 15 or 20 percent have candida in varying degrees.

"Patients with candida should avoid all processed foods, and especially those with sugar, such as soft drinks. Get back to the basics. Grow your own garden if you can. If not, maybe go to a health food store, where you can buy organic, unprocessed foods. While most Americans eat too much fat, people with candida need to be more concerned with sugar than with fat. If you eliminate nutritionally poor foods, you will often be surprised at how your taste for things changes as your diet changes."

Dr. Ray Wunderlich emphasizes the link between depression and such physical imbalances as candidiasis and thyroid disease. "A very high percentage of the people I see who are depressed also have imbalances, such as an overgrowth of candida. Thyroid disease is another example. If you considered all the women whom I treat in my practice, from 70 to 75 percent of them would have thyroid disease, and an even higher percentage would have some form of candida, which is yeast overgrowth.

"A good example is a TV reporter I saw this morning. After

coming into my office to film a segment on my approach to medicine, she got personally interested in what I do. She is 40 years old. We did a mineral analysis on her and found that she is deficient in five nutrient minerals. She is a perfectly normal, functioning individual of 40 years of age. But when you examine her carefully, it turns out that she has recurrent vaginal yeast infections, some bloating, some gas and indigestion, and she has taken antibiotics: a classic profile of a candida patient, which is all too common. In a place like Florida, where the weather is so humid and molds and yeasts grow so readily, problems associated with recurrent yeast infections are almost an epidemic."

Dr. Walt Stoll brings his understanding of the body's immune system to bear on his clinical approach. He describes his clinical experience using examples from candidiasis patients, with references to rheumatoid arthritis patients and others. As he explains: "The immune system sees the world in black and white. Something entering your body that it comes in contact with is either you or it is not you. If it is you, the immune system is not supposed to attack; if it is not you, then it *is* supposed to attack. One of the things that your digestive tract does is to break down things from the environment into particles small enough for you to absorb without alerting your immune system that they came from somewhere else besides you. But if, for example, your gut is not doing the job perfectly, it leaks a particle of protein (a peptide) that is large enough to alert the immune system, in your joints, muscles, or ligaments, for instance. Then your immune system can't tell the difference between the protein particle from outside and the one in your tissues, so it attacks both. Let's imagine that every time you have corn, for example, you don't break it down perfectly and one of those peptides leaks out of your intestine. Your body attacks the corn peptide, but it's also attacking the peptide—that is identical to the corn peptide—in your muscle, ligament, and joint. You'll feel that immune response as arthritis, tendonitis, or other conditions.

"If you stop the process," Dr. Stoll continues, "the immune system settles down in three and a half days, and you begin showing improvement. The first example I heard of was about ten years ago. If you took someone with rheumatoid arthritis or took a group of these patients and put them on a fast, 75 percent of them would improve within a week. You can't keep someone on a water fast forever, of course; but here was a dramatic illustration of the fact that there was another cause of rheumatoid arthritis that we could address. We didn't necessarily have to limit our course of treatment to gold shots, cortisone, and a crippling future for the patients.

"There are a number of things that make the gut more permeable to peptides. Stress is one of them. We know not to go swimming right after we eat, because there is not enough blood supply in the body to adequately supply both the intestinal tract and the muscles. When your blood supply is concentrated in your intestinal tract digesting your meal, going for a vigorous swim risks not getting enough blood in the muscles, resulting in cramps and, possibly, drowning. When you are chronically stressed—and most stresses are not psychological but environmental—your body deals with it with a fight-or-flight response, which makes your muscles get a little more chronically tight and active. Your body concentrates more blood supply into the fight-or-flight area and then takes away the blood supply from the intestinal tract. The intestinal lining replaces itself on average about every 14 hours, so it requires a heavy blood supply. If you are chronically stressed for long enough, eventually the intestinal lining functions less normally, which of course produces other imbalances. The normal bacteria that are supposed to grow sometimes get out of balance and allow candida to move in and flourish. This damages the lining further and so things leak even more.

"I've been practicing medicine with an awareness of these types of problems for 15 years and in my experience this food absorption syndrome is the main cause of brain fatigue, or 'brain fag,' as it is called. By the time I see most of my patients, they have had everything else tried unsuccessfully on them and a large percentage of them have this syndrome as their basic cause. If the patient is willing to follow directions, within a few weeks they already see enough improvement so that they know they are doing the right thing. Within a few months, they've usually improved enough so that they can handle it from there on their own.

"My procedure is to first collect all the medical records that the person has accumulated up to that time, so I don't have to repeat any tests that have already been done. If some things have obviously been missed, then I try to fill in the gaps. There are labs around the country that do a pretty good job of looking for parasites, candidiasis, low magnesium, and other disorders that are either not done or done poorly by conventional labs. I look at the entire chronological history of the patient for a couple of weeks before their appointment and try to think of any factor that might have influenced their health and that might be indicated as a pattern of change over time. Then we have the regular data bases that we use in conventional medicine to look for other kinds of patterns. I'll also ask the patient to keep a record of his or her usual diet and anything special that they ingest for a week or so. Then I put all those pieces together with a general physical exam and see if the pattern suggests some of these other causes.

"Finally, when I get a picture and it's pretty obvious what is happening, I educate the patient sufficiently so that he or she can make an informed decision about going forward with the therapy. I tell patients to make their decision very carefully, so that once having decided to go ahead they then are able to maintain that commitment. That way, we are sure that if the patient doesn't get well it is because we were wrong, and not because the patient was careless about sticking to his or her diet and regimen. Generally, I can predict within a few days how long it is going to take for the person to start feeling better. I have patients keep a record of their symptoms so that they can track their own progress and improvement. As you get better, frequently you forget how badly you were feeling before. Unless someone lives with a patient, it's hard to assess exactly where you are once a patient begins to improve.

"The treatment depends upon the cause, of course. If the person has candidiasis, then the treatment is relatively simple and straightforward. A strict diet is necessary for a while. I will probably have to give them some digestive enzymes to correct the poor protein metabolism, until they can do some relaxation techniques to get the blood supply back to the intestinal tract, which usually takes from three to six months. In the presence of candidiasis, I usually use some Nystatin, a prescription anti-fungal agent, to try to directly attack the candida problem. If the person hadn't been absorbing things too well for a while I might use some concentrated nutrients with antioxidants to try to replenish the body with what it needs to repair itself and to improve the immune function."

"Ellen," "Cynthia," "Nancy," "Bob," and "Jack:" Personal Accounts of Candidiasis

"Ellen"

"I have suffered from chronic candidiasis since I was about 13. We think it might have been linked to my taking massive doses of sulfa drugs for kidney problems when I was younger. I can't remember a time since I was 13—and I'm 31 now—when I didn't have a yeast infection. There may have been two- and three-week periods when I wasn't suffering from symptoms, but I always, to some extent, had a very severe yeast infection. I went to conventional doctors and they gave me the typical vaginal and topical cremes, and basically patted my hand and told me to come back and see them in two weeks. These medications seemed to help during the time that I used them, but invariably the infection returned, and was often twice as bad after I stopped the treatment. So after a while, I simply avoided going to see any physician and just lived with the problem, except on the occasions when my symptoms got so severe that I just had to go see someone.

"Eventually, I went for a Pap smear and a nurse practitioner suggested that I read a book called The Yeast Syndrome. *It wasn't until I read the book and got Dr. Stoll's name out of it that I even connected my physical ailments with my mental health. I had always been moody and prone to periods of depression and there was a history of depression in my family. I never needed to be hospitalized, but I felt that some of these bouts, especially during my adolescent and college years, were extremely severe. I suffered mood swings*

97

and would have described myself as having a very volatile personality. But after going to Dr. Stoll, who started me on oral Nystatin, changed my diet, and used various supplements to correct my nutritional and physiological deficiencies, within about 60 days I felt like a totally different person. In fact, my husband commented that it was like being married to a different person. In hindsight, I can see that as my candidiasis symptoms were eradicated, my mental symptoms disappeared. So I use mental symptoms now as a red flag. If I start seeing personality changes within myself, I take a look at what I've been eating lately and how I've been feeling, and make some changes there. Then I seem to get back on track.

"I have learned that conventional treatments that just treat the symptoms are not going to help you. You have to look for the root cause of your ailments. There is help out there to be found. You simply have to find someone like Dr. Stoll who knows how to treat your illness, and comply with their recommendations. You will get better."

"Cynthia"

"Ever since I began modeling in New York about 15 years ago, I've had tremendous difficulty with depression and also with hypoglycemia, which was then a very fashionable disease. I was constantly on a diet and constantly in doctors' offices for yeast infections and digestive and stomach problems. I visited a lot of doctors who would tell me it was all in my head and send me to psychiatrists. I spent the better part of 20 years going from doctor to doctor

for various things, having my husband tell me that I was a hypochondriac and feeling like one, and also working things out in therapy trying everything that I could until I went to Dr. Stoll.

"In the beginning, Dr. Stoll didn't find out that I had candida. Part of working with Dr. Stoll is learning to take responsibility for your own health, and that was a big switch in my life. Part of my health that was causing me a big problem was dental, so I went and had a lot of dental surgery done and came back to Dr. Stoll sicker than I have ever been in my life, with tremendously severe headaches. I felt as if someone was banging a steel hammer inside my head. And I was angry, even though I had been working with my feelings in therapy. So I wasn't afraid of expressing my feelings, which was good, but I felt angry all the time. Dr. Stoll had me do a stool test, and it came out that I had an abundance of candida. At the time, Dr. Stoll explained to me that when you do dental work, research has shown it will exacerbate candida. In its way, this problem was a gift to me because in the past, I had only half-believed that I had candida. I didn't make a commitment to getting better. This time, within two months after taking Nystatin and vitamins, and doing aerobics, and going to a therapist to make sure that I got everything worked out, I was a different person.

"I felt so totally different that it gave me the perspective to look back over the previous 20 years of my life and say, 'Oh, if only I had known all of this then, I wouldn't have done all of that.' I had spent my life running down the wrong roads. And

it was such a relief because the change allowed me to really begin to live. Now I have my little ritual. I take my vitamins and do my aerobics, and make sure that I keep my house environmentally clean of gases and pollutants that exacerbate the condition. The change in how I felt was like going from 2 percent to 98 percent well. It was so dramatic."

"Nancy"

"My youngest child was born with a lot of health problems—nothing life-threatening, he was just sick all the time. He lived on antibiotics from the day he was born until he was about five years old. He cried all the time and never slept. Most people don't think of an infant as being depressed, but when a baby cries all the time, you could say he's depressed, or in an anxious state, or in a state of pain. It was certainly very stressful for the both of us. As it turned out, most of his problems were allergy-related. He had ear infections, bronchitis, very severe eczema, and his digestive tract had become very permeable.

"Within a month after I had taken my son to Dr. Stoll, and we had begun regenerating his intestinal lining through treating his candidiasis and watching his diet, I began seeing some improvement. Six months later, he was a totally different child. We were a totally different family.

"At that point, I recommended that my mother-in-law go see Dr. Stoll as well, because my child had inherited all these allergy problems from my mother-in-law. She had severe asthma and emphysema, as well as a multitude of other problems. She had gotten

to the point where she was extremely depressed because she thought that she was dying. I think that had I not gotten her to Dr. Stoll, her life would have ended years before it did. She was so sick that she would crawl out of bed in the morning to a chair, and just wheeze and cough all day long in that same chair. She could do no housework, she no longer had a driver's license, and she didn't go anywhere. She spent more time in the hospital than she did at home anyway. He life would have depressed anyone.

"So I took my mother-in-law to Dr. Stoll and within a month or two, she started showing tremendous improvement. Within about four to five months, she was a totally different person. The care she received literally turned her life around. She took the driver's test and got her driver's license again. She bought herself a car and became very active among senior citizens. The depression was gone. This lady just turned around. She now had a totally different personality. She had been on 13 different drugs at the time I took her to Dr. Stoll, for a multitude of problems, and he probably got her off three-fourths of them. Her attitude changed tremendously, just as my youngest child's had."

"Bob"

"I had been sick for 25 years and was just slowly getting worse. At my worst, I passed out and wrecked my car. It was really hard to work and I was getting very depressed. I went to the local doctors, the local hospital, and even tried five days at the Mayo Clinic. They sent me back with sleeping

pills and tranquilizers, and told me that it was all in my head. Finally I went to Dr. Stoll, who was the tenth doctor I'd seen. He read over my history in about five minutes and said, 'Well, I can almost guarantee you that I know what is wrong with you.' He sent off a stool sample, which is an $80 lab test. When it came back, it confirmed his diagnosis. I had candida and giardia, little parasites eating holes in me. I went through this whole process of changing my diet and treating the candida and giardia and in about three months, I got better. I thought I was cured so I started eating the same old junk, and got sick again. I did that about twice. So it really took me about a year to get totally cured. But now it has been about two years and I am completely cured, thanks to Dr. Stoll.

"*Things had gotten so bad. My wife wouldn't leave me and I was dragging her down. I was borrowing money from my family just to keep going and the Mayo Clinic had said that it was all in my head. I had no reason to think that I was ever going to get better and I was continually getting worse. So I decided to commit suicide. And I remembered when I was a kid that our dad always told us, 'Kids, if you ever want to commit suicide, that is okay, but there is only one acceptable method. And that is starvation.' So I said to myself, 'Fine, all I have to do is stop eating for about three months and I will be dead. That sounds real good to me.' So I did. I stopped eating, and of course after about two days of not eating my symptoms went away. At the time I didn't realize that it was the food that I was eating that was contributing to my being so sick and depressed.*

So I got to feeling better and started eating again, and got sick again. To people out there who are really, really depressed and have decided to just chuck it all in, I say, starvation is the only way to commit suicide because you may find that if you stop eating, your symptoms go away. Plus it gives you plenty of time to reconsider.

"No words can describe the joy of living in a healthy body after being sick for a long time. I can now eat almost anything except sugar—meaning sucrose—honey, and potatoes. I can eat fructose, corn syrup, and any other forms of sugar. When I was at the Mayo Clinic, we went through five days of tests and at the end of it I had a list of possibilities. One of those possibilities was food allergies. And I said, 'I'm here, you have this nice big laboratory, why don't you test me for food allergies?' The internist, who acted like the director of the show, got mad. He said, 'You don't have food allergies, and I'm not going to test you for them.' So those are the kind of people I was dealing with at the Mayo Clinic. I have toyed with the idea of going back to the Mayo Clinic or writing them a letter, but I haven't because I'm convinced that they would just put my letter aside and say, 'Oh, another hypochondriac.'

"Dr. Stoll has been persecuted by the Kentucky Medical Board for years for that very reason. Some of his patients went back to their old doctors after they were cured and told them what had been wrong. Some of these other doctors got so embarrassed and mad that they filed charges against Walt Stoll with the Kentucky board. There has never been a patient complaint against him; the only complains were from *other doctors. So going back to your old doctor and explaining can sometimes have very negative repercussions."*

"Jack" (described by "Gail," his wife)

"For ten years my husband suffered with what was diagnosed as acute, chronic gastritis and depression. For a long time, we didn't link the two. So he was treated for gastritis and suffered several endoscopies, and for his depression took lithium, Prozac, you name it. Neither condition got much better. We eventually decided that he should stop taking all those heavy-duty drugs because they seemed to be doing more damage than good. Finally, we heard about Dr. Stoll and he diagnosed my husband as having candidiasis. With the use of the anti-yeast medication Nystatin, and diet and vitamin therapy, he got better on both counts—the gastritis and the depression—very rapidly. We saw a change within about two months.

"We had spent ten years, going from doctor to doctor and hospital to hospital, trying to figure out what was wrong. He had been hospitalized with panic attacks; he had really been put through the mill. After all of that, his treatment and cure turned out to be quite simple."

13. Chronic Fatigue

Today's medical buzzword is chronic fatigue syndrome. This refers to the kind of incredible fatigue that makes people unable to get out of bed in the morning for weeks at a time. Most fatigue-centered conditions begin slowly. A person gradually feels less energized than in prior months or years. They just can't do the things they did before.

As Dr. Allan Spreen tells us, "Physical and emotional fatigue go hand-in-hand. Fatigue tends to affect mental functioning, so that a person suffering from fatigue feels that his or her memory is not as good as it once was. I consider that type of fatigue biochemically based. I'm sure it's in the genes that some people wear out faster than others."

Food sensitivities, fatigue, and mental health are often linked. Turning again to Dr. Spreen: "Food sensitivities often manifest themselves as cravings. We try to get people off the foods they crave. Chances are they may be sensitive to these foods, such that their sensitivity can manifest itself as fatigue and mental states tied to fatigue, such as irritability or frustration.

"Depression is another commonly experienced reaction to

fatigue. People think they're getting old or sick, or that they're dying, because they don't have the energy they once had. And depression causes a domino effect. Once people are depressed they don't care to do anything. If they don't do anything their self-worth decreases. They feel worse and worse.

"We try to take a complete approach. We find that as digestion improves, with proper foods and supplemental digestive enzymes, fatigue tends to diminish. Subsequently, energy levels and clarity of mind improve. People can concentrate better. The patient can remember things better because his or her mind isn't experiencing brain fog from all of the toxic junk floating around in the body.

"We ask people to give us two weeks. We want them to stop eating the foods they crave the most. If there is anything they feel the day just isn't complete without, we tell them that that's what they need to give up first. Once they give that up, if their fatigue worsens for the next two or three days—if they become more irritable, pick fights with family members, their self-worth diminishes, feel like they're not getting anywhere, have more intestinal problems—I can almost guarantee that that food is a major part of their problem.

"Once they get past that hump, which I call withdrawal—the signs of withdrawal described above confirm the presence of a food sensitivity, or allergy, to craved food in question—they tend to feel much better and everything seems to improve. Their peace of mind improves; they are less fatigued; their depression tends to decrease, if it's not true clinical depression from some other cause; their energy level increases; sleep improves; and the quality of their relationships improves. Their state of mind seems to dominate the other way where everything becomes better. It's not a panacea but it's a place to start."

Dr. Spreen outlines a nutritional approach to regaining energy: "Our efforts here are to optimize a person's biochemical intake nutritionally so that he or she can make the best use of whatever genetic disposition they have and overcome fatigue. Of course, there's always the possibility that fatigue represents the onset of something serious like cancer or something else. Our approach to treatment is to consult on a nutritional basis, complementing whatever diagnosis a patient might have from their primary physician. We don't seek to replace a primary physician.

"Normally I start by taking the known stressors out of the diet. The first three are sugar, sugar, and sugar. When people eat a lot of refined sugar, the body tries to bring the sugar level down. Their sugar levels bounce up and down, up and down. They're getting highs and lows, which make their mind fog up and prevent clear thinking and memory.

"This is a frustrating situation. When people get frustrated they get irritated. When they get irritated they pick fights or get depressed. Their self-worth goes down or they hit their wife or smack their kids when they really don't mean to. Sugary items alone are usually a major part of most people's diets and a hard thing to stop.

"After we've taken the refined sugar out of the diet we do other simple things. We ask people to eat foods in their natural state, not processed foods. If a person stays on junk all the time— eats 12 candy bars a day, three soft drinks or more (with seven teaspoons of sugar in each soft drink), and smokes and drinks and gets stimulants in other bad foods—taking a multivitamin just isn't going to do the trick.

"I try to get people off caffeine (found in coffee, soft drinks, and cocoa) and theophylline (found in tea). A person who says,

107

'Gee doc, just don't take away my coffee in the morning,' or 'Don't take away my chocolate,' has just picked the thing that they most need to give up. I don't consider coffee a food. It's a toxin, but since people drink it, we have to consider it a food item.

"I give people vitamins and supplements which, hopefully, their bodies will absorb. If their absorption is not good they may require digestive enzymes, additional acidophilus, or hydrochloric acid supplements."

Finally, Dr. Spreen emphasizes two naturally occurring substances as being of particular importance in the treatment of chronic fatigue: "We find that people straighten out to a large degree if they straighten out what goes into their mouth. And it's rewarding. Two of the types of nutrients we use to overcome fatigue are the following:

* "B Vitamins. I almost always recommend that a person with fatigue start with a B_{12} shot, the old 'quack' remedy that most doctors consider a placebo and don't even like to talk about. I try to get a B_{12} shot into anybody that mentions fatigue because it's cheap, harmless, and easy, and the results are so good. I'm batting about three out of four that just with a B_{12} shot you'll feel more energy within a day.

"B complex is needed today more than ever before in the American diet. The foods most of us eat are almost totally refined. Most of our carbohydrates have been processed, resulting in nutrient loss. All of the B vitamins work together, predominantly to help with the assimilation of carbohydrates. When complex carbohydrates are removed from the diet, people use up their B complex stores in the body, which are somewhat limited, being water-soluble. If people consumed more unrefined foods, they would have what is required in the food for the assimilation of that food. So I give both B complex in a supplement and extra B_{12} if fatigue is a problem. Plus I try to get people off refined sugar, refined white flour, refined pasta, and anything else that might stress the body.

> * "Herbs. I'm not an herbalist but I'm using herbs more and more in my practice. To boost mental function, I use ginkgo biloba, probably the number-two herb after ginseng. We'll give a trial of that to people who say they don't remember things the way they used to, and to children with learning disorders. We'll try the herb for about six weeks. If the person doesn't feel a noticeable difference in that time we'll conclude that it probably doesn't work for them. The nice thing about this type of remedy is that it's harmless. If it doesn't work, you've only lost a few dollars; it hasn't done any harm. I tend to think that herbs with a 2,000-year history have done people some good.

"Some botanicals that worry us are at the opposite end of the spectrum. We want to get these substances out of the body. Nonherbal teas and coffee bother us because they are artificial stimulants. They make people feel good momentarily but harm them in the long run. We compare it to the difference between feeding a horse right and whipping a horse. You can make a horse work harder for awhile with the whip, but you'd better feed him or he won't continue to work. We try to get the whips out of there and enhance nutrition instead.

"If we can help a person sleep we can help him or her to think and feel better when awake. Valerian is an herb that has been used for years to help with sleep. Sometimes we mix that with taurine, which is not an herb but an amino acid. These two agents together tend to help people relax, although this does not work all the time.

"This combination is not nearly as good as tryptophan, which was removed from the market a few years ago. There was a really shameful campaign to have it removed by people who claimed tryptophan caused a toxicity reaction. But the toxic reactions had nothing to do with pure tryptophan at all. Tryptophan produced wonderful results. It was the best help for depression, sleep disorders, and mood swings. But I understand that tryptophan is still available out of this country.

"There are a lot of herbals that help to alleviate individual complaints. Although my expertise with herbs is still limited, I'm finding them increasingly helpful in my practice. I think that herbalists past and present, dating back to the Indian medicine men and ancient Chinese herbalists, knew what they were doing."

14. Hormone Imbalance

Emphasizing the importance of having access to good testing facilities, Dr. Ray Wunderlich cites the importance of hormone imbalances among the illnesses that are often misdiagnosed as mental disease. "When we assess people's hormones and glandular functions with good chemistry, we can help make them less sensitive to the toxic assaults of the environment.

"While there are no such things as panaceas in medicine and we want to beware of unwarranted enthusiasm and zeal," Dr. Wunderlich continues, "the hormone DHEA is probably the closest thing to a panacea in medicine that we have found as of yet. It is the so-called 'mother hormone' of the adrenal gland, an antidepressant that seems to be able to counter a lot of the allergic reactions that we see in people who are accumulating toxic insults as they age, decade after decade. This adrenal hormone declines from the age of 20 to death, due to illness and aging. By intervening with appropriate doses of the adrenal hormone DHEA, we can reverse many of the allergies and immune susceptibilities that we see in people over 25 years of age.

"Mental functioning is also impaired in people who are low in the adrenal hormones, especially in DHEA. When these hormones are down, people become chronically fatigued. They have difficulty getting into mental gear, making decisions, seeing options, and fighting off the chemical assaults found in their environment. We can measure adrenal function in the saliva and the blood, and we can show that it increases with DHEA supplementation.

"Here's a typical case that I have treated. A 40-year-old woman was having marital difficulties and had been seeing a counselor for a couple of years for this problem. While she did need to straighten out her interpersonal relationship, that wasn't causing her physical and emotional problems. She was deficient in adrenal hormone. She was tired and irritable and couldn't get through the day. She couldn't manage the children. They would get on her nerves and she'd fire off at her husband. I tested her blood level of DHEA and found that it was more than two standard deviations below the mean. I put her on a very minimal dose of DHEA, and within two or three months she had discharged all of her counselors and her husband called me to tell me what saviors we were. These are some of the miracles we see.

"Not every case is going to be a miracle cure. But some cases of chronic depression, irritability, and premenstrual syndrome are related to adrenal dysfunction, with low levels of the mother hormone of the adrenal gland. This is particularly so in people with low-blood-sugar symptoms.

"We believe that this DHEA is kind of a baseline hormone. It feeds all the other systems, including the ones that regulate the sugar balance in the body. It can also serve as a precursor to the sex hormones—both female and male—as well as to the electrolytes, the salt and water hormones of the adrenals. It is highly individual in its response, but it is a major reactor that we didn't know about some years ago. The effects of DHEA have been well-researched; it has an anti-cancer, anti-viral, and anti-depressive effect in animals. People have improved through the use of herbs, vitamins, and minerals, which have probably been supporting the functioning of this hormone in the body, among other effects.

"People who are tired when they get up in the morning, who have reactions to sugar, who have to eat frequent meals, who have family histories of low blood sugar, diabetes, or alcoholism, and those with stubborn allergies," Dr. Wunderlich concluded, "frequently have low adrenal function. Vitamins and herbs that help support the adrenal function and the precursors of the adrenal function are vitamin C, pantothenic acid, B-complex, licorice, and Siberian ginseng."

15. Nutrient Imbalances in the Body and Brain

Dr. Priscilla Slagle has made a unique and important contribution in her medical practice using amino acid supplements to help patients control their mood illnesses by correcting nutrient imbalances in the body and brain. "I have had a lot of clinical experience controlling moods by using amino acids. Right now, I am quite concerned about the current effort by the FDA to ban amino acids, which takes away the right of individuals to help themselves. In a sense, it's like banning proteins, which is to say, ludicrous. So I hope that people will fight this reactionary effort on the part of our government to make amino acids available only through physicians—which would cost a person far more.

"I have treated patients with amino acids for almost 20 years to control moods, for depression, anxiety, memory loss, and other health problems. I continue to be amazed at their efficacy. I usually use them in combination with proper diagnosis and treatment of other conditions.

"The first step I take with my patients is to make the

correct diagnosis. Usually, by the time people get to me, they have already been many places and tried many drugs, and I am the end of the road for them. So these patients don't have simple, straightforward kinds of problems. They usually have multiple-system problems, for instance, chemical sensitivities, viruses, food sensitivities, auto-immune problems, parasite problems, fungus problems, and so on.

"So first I find out what is going on. When a patient comes to me, I often do an amino acid panel so that I can measure 42 different aspects of amino acids in their body. There are 22 amino acids, but I am also measuring metabolic breakdown products. Their patterns suggest connective tissue or auto-immune disease, chronic viruses, chemical or food sensitivities, or candida. While it is an extensive diagnostic process, it does seem to find the root cause of some very puzzling complex physical and mental problems which patients are experiencing.

"Then I remove the offending agents, such as chemicals or candida- or yeast-inducing foods, or drugs (many people have drug-induced auto-immune problems). We have to clarify and clean up their environments and their diets.

"For depression, I use tyrosine, which is an amino acid that raises norepinephrine, a major brain chemical that maintains good mood, drive, motivation, and concentration. Glutamine makes glutamic acid, one of the two major brain fuels, and is important for memory, focus, and concentration. I use these two amino acids to treat depression. They must be combined with the active form of B_6, which controls the absorption, metabolism, and conversion of amino acids into all their various end products, such as neurotransmitters, antibodies, digestive enzymes, muscles, and tissues in the body.

"I also give my depressed patients a basic multivitamin with minerals. Many depressed people are magnesium-deficient, so I've been using a relatively large amount of magnesium in my practice. I've also incorporated a fair amount of potassium for chronic fatigue syndrome patients. Many of them have potassium problems that are not necessarily picked up by a standard blood test. I check cellular potassium levels rather than the regular blood tests. I use some homeopathic cortisone with certain people with auto-immune disease.

"Some other amino acids that I use are taurine and cysteine. Taurine is a neuro-inhibitory neurotransmitter which has a calming effect. It also controls heart rate and helps with fat metabolism. Many of the people who have chemical sensitivities and yeast problems (probably 90 percent of the ones I see) have a reduced taurine as well as a reduced cysteine level. Cysteine, like taurine, is an amino acid that helps the body to detoxify.

"In many people with chemical sensitivities, the detoxification processes in their bodies has broken down due to overload, or deficiencies of various nutrients, or a liver dysfunction. So they aren't able to handle the same kind of toxic load that other people might handle who aren't dealing with the same variables. I use large doses of vitamin C and multi-amino acids, as well as certain other products which support detoxification pathways.

"At the risk of sounding fanatical, I believe we are poisoning this earth. Many people with chemical sensitivities, auto-immune disorders, and immune deficiency problems are early victims of what is happening to the planet, harbingers of what may later grow into a more serious and more obviously recognized problem. I have begun to see in my practice a vast number of auto-immune problems that I feel are environmentally or chemically induced. This problem is significant and deserves to receive national and international attention. I really appreciate the work that Dr. Rodgers has done and I recommend that people, particularly those with chemical sensitivities, read her books."

Dr. Sidney Baker emphasizes magnesium deficiency in his clinical practice when treating nutrient imbalances that manifest as mental disease. "I presented a paper on magnesium at a conference in La Jolla, California, a few years ago. At this colloquium, there were magnesium experts from all over, mostly academic people, and mostly people who had jobs like running an intensive care unit or a cardiac care unit, or a department of immunology or obstetrics and gynecology. Everyone there from every medical specialty was saying, 'Isn't it amazing that our colleagues are not aware of the very lengthy published information on the prevalence of magnesium deficiency in America, and its very widespread picture in clinical practice?' Any ordinary person would have come away from the conference saying, 'Well, how come this problem is being overlooked?' The cynical answer may be the truth: Magnesium deficiency research has no corporate sponsor.

"I've become convinced that magnesium deficiency is a major epidemic, one that we are experiencing right now in North America. Magnesium deficiency is widespread in its pattern of symptoms. It affects cardiovascular disease, allergies, tension, panic attacks, premenstrual syndrome, and hyperactivity in children, to name just some of the conditions. The underlying theme behind many of the symptoms is what you might call being 'uptight.'

"Both magnesium and yeast problems probably began around 1950. The magnesium problem probably has its roots in the widespread use in agriculture of fertilizers containing potassium. The yeast problem probably arose because of the widespread use of antibiotics in the population, which began around 1950.

"Many people come to see me specifically because they think that I am a yeast specialist, and so perhaps I see these patients in disproportionate numbers. But I think that this epidemic, which is being disregarded by many people in mainstream medicine, is simply overwhelming in its prevalence in the United States. Many people's medical histories show a quite obvious yeast problem. They started getting sick soon after they started taking antibiotics; they have bloating and difficulty concentrating; they have intolerances to foods, gastrointestinal disturbances, and recurring vaginitis. Unfortunately, when they seek help from most doctors, they are told, 'Gee, we're very skeptical about this whole yeast idea; it isn't proven and so therefore we won't put you on simple remedies to see if you might have it.' The dogma has overcome the simple observation of nature.

"As a practitioner, I have a worm's-eye view of the world. I see things very close to nature and hear from my patients directly about what is going on with their health. I have formed strong opinions that these epidemics—magnesium deficiency, problems with fatty acids or yeast, calcium and trace mineral deficiencies—are keys to people's health and well-being, both in terms of finding good preventive measures and in terms of finding cures. It is very dangerous when people who are intelligent and strong-willed get themselves into positions of authority within the medical bureaucracy, and feel quite justified in dictating what they consider to be the truth, rather than letting the truth grow, in an organic way, from the experience of those of us who are seeing patients."

Dr. Lendon Smith has also confirmed the importance of

the magnesium factor, both in his clinical practice and in research studies in both animals and humans. "I've been working with a chemist out of Spokane, Washington, whose name is John Kitkoski. He started doing experiments with horses by taking blood samples and then testing for mineral and other nutrient deficiencies. He discovered that some of these horses were low in calcium, or magnesium, for example. So he would put standard feed out in the corral, and then he would put standard feed plus calcium, or magnesium, or zinc, and let the animals go out and freely eat. They would smell everything and eat only what they needed. If they were low in calcium, they would eat just the calcium-supplemented feed, and then when they had had enough he noticed that they would come back to the standard feed. He would take a blood test and find out that their body chemistry had returned to normal. He figured out that the reason why the nose is placed in front of the mouth is to tell us 'don't eat that' or 'do eat this.' The sense of smell, along with taste, is a monitoring system.

"With hundreds of hours of data to verify his hypothesis, Mr. Kitkoski and I have found that people who are low in magnesium are more likely to have emotional problems—to experience anxiety and tension, to be upset, and to be unable to relax in sleep—and that leads to secondary factors. If the body chemistry is balanced, then the body can handle almost any kind of stress or stressors that come along. If it is not, then stress can exacerbate the problem.

"Mr. Kitkoski also noticed that 80 percent of the people living in North America—and he has enough data to verify this—are somewhat alkaline. If the body is alkaline, then minerals are not soluble enough to make the enzymes do their job.

"The way to determine the levels of chemicals in your body

is to have blood tests done. If the GGT level is low, a person is low in magnesium because it's a magnesium-run enzyme. If a person has high levels of GGT, they often have too much magnesium. Mr. Kitkoski uses the standard 0 to 40 to 50 on the testing, going by the deviation from the mean. If somebody has around 20 on their GGT, then they are probably alright. But if they are low, and they have signs of anxiety and tension, if they can't relax, get spooked by people, and can't seem to handle the stresses of the world, then magnesium will help."

16. Premenstrual Syndrome (PMS)

Dr. Hyla Cass emphasizes how often biochemical imbalances and psychological problems coexist. In her practice, she combines her work as a holistic psychiatrist with her awareness of and use of naturally occurring substances to restore biochemical balance. A good example of how this approach can work is in the treatment of premenstrual syndrome. Dr. Cass describes a typical case: "A 30-year-old woman came to see me recently, two months after she had broken up with her boyfriend. She was depressed. She'd gained weight. She was exhausted. She had trouble keeping up with her work as a secretary. Psychotherapy wasn't helping. I asked her what she was eating and it turned out that there were a number of dietary patterns that were contributing to her emotional state.

"I took a careful history which revealed that, while she wasn't overeating, she had developed the habit of drinking coffee and eating sweets to counter fatigue. Not only did this cause her to gain weight, but the coffee and sweets induced a hypoglycemic cycle. Her blood sugar levels were irregular, and this caused her to feel anxious. It was as though at a certain time of the day she was going into a withdrawal phase and the caffeine and sugar would help bring her back up.

"So the first part of her problem was this hypoglycemic cycle. Her other problem was PMS, which had grown worse over the past few months. Her symptoms included mood swings, irritability, water retention, craving sweets, and weight gain. She had always thought that PMS was normal, that this was what women (and their hapless partners) had to live with—a misconception held by too many women.

"Her lab work revealed that she did have a fairly low fasting blood sugar level. To handle the hypoglycemia, I prescribed a specific diet and supplement program. For the PMS, I recommended the following regiment: For the first two weeks of her cycle, a dong quai herbal combination; then for the second two weeks, a specific PMS combination containing extra vitamin B_6, magnesium, and ingredients that detoxify the liver, an important component in treating PMS. (The specific ZAND herbal formulas are particularly effective.) I also recommended regular exercise.

"After a month on this regimen, she was feeling much, much better. She started to feel like she had some control over the break-up with her boyfriend and over her work problems. She was able to take control of her problems rather than allowing these factors in her life to control her.

"This was one case of depression where psychotherapy alone simply was not enough. What she really needed was psychotherapy plus the combination of herbal and natural remedies, diet, and exercise.

"In cases where this nutritional regimen is not sufficient, I prescribe natural progesterone cream from day 14 until day 28 of the menstrual cycle. The kind of progesterone I recommend is a natural progesterone, not the progesterone that's in the regular pharmaceutical birth control pills or the hormones that are administered by prescription. It's a derivative from the wild Mexican yam and is available in health food stores. It's also useful for menopausal symptoms. It is applied topically to the skin on fatty areas of the body, where it can be easily absorbed." Hormonal imbalance can be corrected naturally. The following case, also from Dr. Hyla Cass, is another example.

"Not long ago, a 48-year-old woman came in to see me complaining that her life 'just wasn't working.' She was a very successful professional. She had a great marriage. Her children were grown and in college and they were doing well. Her husband was successful. She really had a very good life, and yet she was unhappy. Now you could simply call this a mid-life crisis, and do psychotherapy.

"However, when I took a psychological history, aware that this was a time of life for her to start looking inward, to evaluate her life, at the same time I asked her about her menstrual cycles. She said she was still menstruating. Her periods were changing in frequency and amount, but with no other symptoms. I sent her to the lab and it turned out she was very low in progesterone, low in estrogen, but particularly low in progesterone.

"I prescribed the natural progesterone cream, which helped to alleviate most of her psychological symptoms. Her irritability went way down. She realized that her uneasiness was metabolically based. It wasn't simply a personal psychological issue. She was peri-menopausal.

"Hormonal changes occur subtly over time, and peri-menopausal women will often think that their problems are purely psychological in origin. They will not think to look at what's going on biochemically in the body. Aside from the progesterone cream, I also prescribed the herbal formulas, which improved her condition even further."

Dr. Cass concludes: "Even though people do have psychological issues—and it is important to deal with them—it's equally important to look at and treat the underlying chemistry. Often the psychological problems will lessen in severity or even disappear with treatment of biochemical imbalances."

Dr. Doris Rapp emphasizes the part food cravings can play in the development of premenstrual syndrome. "The foods that you crave premenstrually are the foods that could be causing you to feel sick. I know one mother whose premenstrual chocolate cravings were so powerful that she would put the chocolate bars in the freezer to at least slow down the pace at which she would eat them when she was premenstrual. If you are a chocoholic and you can't manage without eating chocolate, it's a good bet that chocolate is a food that is causing you a problem."

17. Thyroid Disorders

The thyroid gland is a very important component of the immune system. It is, as Dr. Hyla Cass describes it, "the energy-generating gland located below the Adam's apple in the neck." Dr. Cass emphasizes the importance of thyroiditis as a root cause of a variety of emotional and physical problems. She also describes difficulties today in establishing the diagnosis of thyroid disorder in the face of continuing skepticism from conventional physicians. According to Dr. Cass, "When the thyroid isn't working properly, the immune system is impaired, and this sets up a vicious cycle. You have a person whose immune system is depleted and who is anxious; they're told by regular doctors that the problem is all in their head, that there's nothing physically wrong with them. So then they feel worse.

"I recently saw a young woman who came in depressed, tired, unable to get up on the morning, and feeling overwhelmed by her work responsibilities. Her history revealed that she was often cold, especially in her hands and feet (she even wore socks to bed), had thinning hair, dry skin, constipation, and was losing the outer part of her eyebrows. I suspected an imbalance in her thyroid. When I asked about thyroid disease, she said that it had been suspected before, but her tests had been normal. I checked her thyroid hormones, including thyroid antibody levels.

"Often despite 'normal' blood tests, there is an underactive thyroid. Dr. Broda Barnes' technique of monitoring thyroid function through body temperature is used by many alternative practitioners. Although this patient's thyroid hormone blood levels were normal, she did, in fact, have antithyroid antibodies, confirming a diagnosis of Hashimoto's thyroiditis. This is an auto-immune disease, treatable with thyroid hormone, antioxidants, and adrenal support. Her signs were those of hypothyroidism, indicating that the circulating hormone was being rendered ineffective. With Hashimoto's thyroiditis, there are often also intermittent signs of hyperthyroidism, or overactive thyroid, such as irritability or heart palpitations.

"I prescribed thyroid hormone from natural (animal) sources, and asked her to monitor her body temperature, so I could adjust the dosage. She asked whether this supplementation would suppress her own thyroid function, and whether she would be taking it for the rest of her life. The answer was 'no' on both counts. The treatment actually supported her own gland, allowing it to heal. Within ten days of starting the program she was feeling alive again.

"A surprisingly large number of patients that I see have thyroiditis. I really can't emphasize the importance of this problem enough because thyroiditis often accompanies the mixed infection syndrome, which can consist of any combination of the following: parasites, candida, and the viral syndromes—including the Epstein-Barr virus and the cytomegalo virus. Psychological components include depression, anxiety and even panic attacks.

"To treat thyroiditis, I've done nutritional consults on people that were under the care of other physicians. When I suggested that they had thyroiditis and that it was to be treated with low doses of thyroid hormones, I was met with skepticism from the other doctors.

"When people have these long-standing chronic conditions, they can become extremely depressed. They feel like they can't go on anymore, particularly when their body has been so wracked by the continuing illness. Also, some of the mixed infection of thyroiditis and the parasites or other viruses can actually affect the brain directly. Thyroiditis and its accompanying infections affect the central nervous system along with every other organ of the body. So people come in extremely depressed, both as a reaction to their prolonged illness and as a primary symptom of the illness—and this is usually totally overlooked. That's why it's crucial to do a good medical work-up on a patient whose disorder may at first appear purely psychological in origin," Dr. Cass concludes.

Dr. Stephen Langer asserts that "Many people come into my office with an organic kind of illness that has been misdiagnosed as being either psychosomatic or primarily psychological. Very rarely do I see a patient who comes in with complaints that are primarily psychological in cause. Very often, their complaints have some organic basis which, if taken care of, allows them to resolve much more easily whatever psychological problems they do have.

"The thyroid gland is a little butterfly-shaped organ at the base of the neck that puts out a teaspoon of hormone a year which affects the metabolism and acts as a cellular carburetor for every cell in the body—from our hair follicles down to our toenails. As such, the thyroid can be implicated in just about any kind of condition you can think of. As for its relationship to psychological disorders, since it plays a role in the metabolism of the nervous system, people who have thyroid disorders have conditions like depression, anxiety, panic attacks, and bipolar disorders.

"If a person's metabolism is hypo-functioning, everything is going to be slow. In a book I wrote called *Solve the Riddle of Illness*, I explain why upwards of 40 percent of the population may have subclinical hypothyroidism and not detect it by the traditional blood chemistry work that's done at their general practitioner's office. The symptoms of low thyroid include weakness, dry coarse skin, slow speech, coarse hair, hair loss, weight gain, difficulty breathing, problems with menstruation, nervousness, heart palpitations, brittle nails, and severe chronic fatigue and depression.

"Now if you get somebody with a constellation of symptoms like that they're going to be sick and tired of feeling sick and tired. Plus they're going to feel depressed all the time because they're going from one doctor to another, sometimes with two or three or four pages worth of complaints, and the doctors tell them it's all in their head, or that they should go home and learn to live with it. Obviously you're going to see depression. Now not everything that I see is hypothyroidism by any means. But hypothyroidism is so easy to identify and so ubiquitous in the population, and it can be treated so well and so rapidly for so little money, that it's become a primary interest of mine.

"To treat someone with hypothyroidism, I put them on as little as a quarter of a grain, which is a newborn-infant dose, and this produces a radical change in the way the person functions. Of course, for someone who has low thyroid function, I also use orthomolecular nutrition and a lot of clinical ecology techniques along with treating the thyroid gland.

"Recently I treated a patient who was the wife of a doctor and the mother of two young children. She basically came in and told me that she didn't want to go on living. She was so tired all the time, and so depressed, that she couldn't keep her head off the pillow after two o'clock in the afternoon. If she didn't go to bed, she would just fall apart. I did a history and physical on her and we made some dietary changes, but basically this woman was profoundly hypothyroid. We put her on a quarter of a grain of thyroid, which is what I start my patients with before building them up very gradually. A quarter of a grain is the smallest dose available. It's such a small quantity that most pharmacies don't even carry it, because when doctors order thyroid they don't even think to order so small a dose. But a quarter of a grain of thyroid was enough. Within a three-week period, this woman not only regained her mental health, but she was out taking tennis lessons, which was shocking even to me because although the treatment usually works it usually takes a longer period of time. So, just that amount of metabolic support was enough to turn this person's life around.

"Another person I treated was a 62-year-old woman who was a member of the Catholic clergy. She had been a nun for at least 30 years when I met her and I will never forget this woman. She came in bloated, profoundly depressed, and fatigued. The only thing that kept her going was basically overworking her adrenal glands. She came in and told me that when she was 12 years old, she went under a dark cloud. When I saw her it was 50 years later, and by that time she had been through 30 or 40 different doctors, including internists, endocrinologists, psychiatrists, and psychologists of various sorts. One of the first things that showed up in her—which I thought was a very positive sign—was that she was freezing all the time. When we did a basal body temperature on her, it never went above 95 degrees. Basal body temperature is a person's resting temperature when she wakes up in the morning. However, when I did a blood work-up on her, all her thyroid hormone levels were within normal limits. I empirically placed her on a dose of thyroid that we gradually built up to about four grains a day, which is quite a high dosage. She's one of the few people I've treated who has needed that high an amount. Within three months her depression of 50 years duration was totally gone.

"Now, obviously she was bitter and angry that she had been suffering for all that time. But the organic feeling that she had of overwhelming fatigue totally disappeared within a three-month period of time, and I've seen that response in thousands of patients over the years. A small dose of thyroid, combined with things like nutritional support and eliminating food allergies, can really turn a person's life around.

"Very often people who are thyroid deficient will have tests that show up normal. It's become apparent, particularly over the past ten years, that some people with thyroid conditions have normal thyroid hormone levels and are suffering from another condition known as Hashimoto's disease, or auto-immune thyroiditis. There is a very precise blood test that any doctor can order called the auto-immune thyroid antibody test, and most of the people who I suspect have thyroid conditions and have normal thyroid hormone levels will have an elevation in their anti-thyroid antibodies. If they have an elevated anti-thyroid antibody level, they have the symptoms that go along with low thyroid, which can be any one of 125 symptoms that we enumerate in *Solve the Riddle of Illness*.

"A lot of the symptoms of thyroiditis are psychological symptoms, such as profound depression. With thyroiditis people get anxiety attacks and panic attacks for no apparent reason. They could be sitting and reading a book. All of a sudden they will develop a cascade of heart palpitations and fearfulness. I've had a number of patients who have been rushed, almost on a monthly basis, to the emergency room to be worked up by cardiologists because their heart was pounding over 200 beats a minute. Cardiologists would do EKG's and echocardiograms and tell them to go see a psychiatrist who would work them up, not find anything, and then put them on an antidepressant or a tranquilizer, and actually make the condition worse. When you have an undiscovered organic basis for a psychological problem, being put on psychotropic medication is like sitting on a thumbtack and being put on pain pills for the rest of your life. It has about the same effect. It wears the system down, and as a result the patient's condition not only does not improve but will in fact deteriorate, because the underlying cause is not being treated.

"To treat patients with thyroiditis, I put them on a trial dose of thyroid and continue to monitor their thyroid hormone levels. Most of these people wind up taking between one and two grains of thyroid a day and their thyroid hormone levels still stay normal despite the fact that their levels were supposedly normal to begin with. More importantly, they get a complete remission of symptoms, many of which manifest themselves as psychological symptoms.

"One woman I treated became a pioneer in the holistic health movement up in northern California. She was in her late 30's and she had exactly the same symptoms that I enumerated above. She had a relatively good job, a stable marriage, and children in school who were no problem, but she was having problems periodically with palpitations and fearfulness, ranging from anxiety to full-blown panic attacks. This woman would call her husband, who was an executive in a large corporation, at least twice a month to tell him that she was having one of the attacks, and he would have to drop everything, come home, and take her to the hospital where she was worked up by psychiatrists and cardiologists who could never find anything. She was, in fact, on a number of different psychotropic medications when she came to see me, in desperation, after reading my book.

"I did a full blood work-up on this woman, and all of her lab tests, with the exception of her anti-thyroid antibodies, were within normal limits. It turned out she did have severe auto-immune thyroiditis. Since her thyroid turned out to be enlarged, we did another test called a thyroid scan, a test that tracks iodine uptake over a 24-hour period and is administered by a radiologist at the hospital. It turned out that her thyroid condition was so severe that she required an operation to remove part of her thyroid—a procedure that is very drastic and is rarely ever indicated. As soon as the operation was done and this woman was placed on a therapeutic diet with the proper nutritional support and a small amount of thyroid, she never had the psychological symptoms again. She went on to become an advocate for holistic and environmental health and founded an organization called the Environmental Health Network which now has thousands of members, including many prominent clinicians. This is an example of how turning one person's life around can affect the lives of many other people.

"The constellation of problems associated with thyroid disorders occurs not only in middle-aged people but also in young people, and not only in women, but also in men. While thyroid disease, particularly auto-immune thyroiditis, is classically considered to be primarily a disease of women, this is just not true. I have seen as many men as women who are suffering from auto-immune thyroiditis and, I might add, from hypothyroidism. Men are really given short shrift and aren't even given the requisite diagnostic tests in many instances to rule out thyroid disease because the medical profession thinks that this is strictly a woman's disorder.

"Moreover, I have seen teenagers and children who are acting out, who are written off as hyperactive, when they may be suffering from a thyroid disorder. Very young children or teenagers express their emotions differently from adults. Sometimes they get written off as being mentally retarded or having minimal brain dysfunction. Then they're given any one of a number of different drugs and placed in special classes. Many times, these young people have thyroid disorders that can be easily treated. But because thyroid dysfunction often leads to frequent infections, these kids are placed on antibiotics. Then they wind up with an overgrowth of yeast in their gut that in turn causes a low-grade inflammation in their gastrointestinal system. As a result, they don't adequately digest their food, so the body starts regarding the food as a foreign invader and puts out antibodies to the food. The child starts exhibiting the classic symptoms of food allergies, which are psychiatric complaints: anxiety attacks, depression, forgetfulness, inability to concentrate, even full-blown panic attacks. In a lot of these cases, you can actually isolate and eliminate the foods that cause an anxiety attack, but merely removing the food is not enough to get to the underlying cause of the disorder. Frequently patients have food allergies because of a pre-existing condition in their digestive systems which has to be addressed. The presence of such a pre-existing condition can cause immune system alterations which result in auto-immune dysfunction. So this is a vicious circle.

133

One of the chief target organs of auto-immune dysfunction is the thyroid gland. You get auto-immune thyroiditis.

"The question for holistic clinicians to ask themselves, regarding each individual patient, is where they're going to intervene. Different physicians will intervene at different places, depending upon their background and interests. I try, to the best of my ability, to get to the root cause of what's going on. If I am having difficulty figuring out the cause, then I try to intervene at a point in a person's imbalance that will cause the least disruption to their lifestyle and give them the best results for the least amount of money in the quickest period of time. Frequently, that turns out to be treating with small doses of thyroid and altering eating habits. In my clinical experience, I have found that with the thyroid and nutritional support, very often a person will get better. The thyroid is not a lifetime treatment and can be removed after the person's condition has been stabilized. Thyroid treatment is inexpensive, works rapidly, and when done properly it is absolutely nontoxic.

"There is one more connection to be drawn between depression and the thyroid dysfunction," Dr. Langer adds: "poor libido. One of the classic symptoms of depression is a loss of interest in sex. Those people who in the past were sexually active, but who all of a sudden or gradually started to lose interest in sex, will be diagnosed as being depressed right away. Men come into my office by the score—many of them young—who have potency problems, and they can't figure it out because they have no apparent organic illness. As a result, they get performance anxiety, and if that continues long enough, they wind up getting severely depressed. But I have found that if you go to the root cause of their depression, very often it's the thyroid that's malfunctioning.

"If a person develops an acute depression that leads to a sexual dysfunction—which it frequently does—a doctor would be remiss if he or she didn't look for an imbalance in the thyroid. Patients have got to start taking their health destinies into their own hands and demanding that doctors do thyroid testing and look for auto-immune thyroid disorders and nutritional imbalances, which are frequently the underlying causes of sexual dysfunction and depression.

"Sleep disturbances are very common with auto-immune thyroiditis. Most people with thyroiditis spend an overwhelming portion of the day in a condition somewhat like low thyroid, which means they're very, very sluggish. The symptoms of thyroiditis include: profound fatigue, memory loss manifested by problems with recent memory and concentration, depression, and nervousness ranging from mild anxiety to full-blown panic attacks. What's really going on is that these people are swinging from low thyroid to high thyroid.

"What triggers an auto-immune response? Imagine auto-immune thyroiditis to be like rheumatoid arthritis of the thyroid gland. A person can have rheumatoid arthritis, which is an auto-immune condition where the body puts out antibodies to the joints. Frequently people with rheumatoid arthritis stay in long periods of remission. When they are under a great deal of stress, the body puts out antibodies to the joints and all their joints swell up. Similarly with the thyroid, if a person gets stressed out for any reason whatsoever, the body can start pumping out antibodies to the thyroid gland. The thyroid becomes acutely inflamed and the hormone which should not be in the system starts escaping. The clinical term for the gland is an 'escaping gland.' The hormone escapes from the gland and it's almost like pumping speed into your system. For some reason (possibly having to do with the cyclical variations in hormone output called diurnal variations), it happens very frequently that people with thyroiditis have an auto-immune reaction at night, making the body put out antibodies, and these people will wake up with their minds racing, their hearts pounding, and feeling anxious and nervous. The problem is often written off as just a sleep disorder—sleep apnea or some sleep problem of unknown cause—when in fact its cause can be detected and corrected," Dr. Langer concludes.

Dr. Allan Spreen reminds us that while thyroid supplementation is an important modality, it is not fail-safe. "I'd love to say that correcting thyroid function is a panacea. While it doesn't work 100 percent of the time, if a patient comes in complaining of fatigue and depression that is linked with the physical findings of foods not digesting well, and cold extremities, then an underactive thyroid may be the root cause. People come and say, 'Oh, my husband says, Don't touch me with your feet at night because they're just ice cold.' These are the same people who are comfortable in a room when everybody else is boiling and they're freezing in a room when everybody else is comfortable. Their thinking seems to have slowed down, they just don't seem to be able to concentrate like they used to, and they don't remember lists the way they used to.

"In this kind of a situation, once I find that their blood levels of thyroid are normal, I go back to the old school of Broda Barnes, who, 40 or 50 years ago, did axillary temperature testing. I ask my patients to keep a record of their early morning basal body temperature. If their basal metabolic rate based on early-morning body temperatures is really low, then I consider them to be candidates for thyroid supplementation. In axillary testing, Broda Barnes talked about temperature ranges between 97.8

and 98.2 degrees Fahrenheit, which is lower than the 98.6 people think of as normal. But the axillary temperature is taken in the armpit first thing in the morning, using a mercury thermometer that stays there for ten minutes before they get up. If their temperature is, much of the time, down in the 96.8, 96.7, 96.5 range, I at least consider the possibility that the person needs low doses of natural thyroid, which is still available.

"Thyroid is a prescription drug, but it can be broken down into very low doses. Some doctors who use this type of testing use synthetic thyroid. I prefer to prescribe natural thyroid in very low doses. If a person responds—either their temperature rises or their symptoms lift—then I retest them to see if their blood levels of thyroid have changed. Many times a person with this profile of symptoms who takes thyroid will feel better, and their blood tests will have remained unchanged, including their thyroid stimulating hormone and their actual thyroid hormone levels. So the blood testing has missed the diagnosis, and yet the person feels well with the increased, but undetectable dose of thyroid hormone."

"Jenny" and "Helen:" Personal Accounts of Thyroiditis

"Jenny"

"I came to be treated by Dr. Spreen only after first following the conventional route in medical treatment. In 1988, I was in my fifth year of infertility treatments, had taken multiple infertility drugs, and wound up severely depressed, which caused me to lose 35 pounds in two months. I couldn't sleep, I had panic attacks, the whole horrible group of

137

symptoms associated with depression. The doctors put me on the conventional Xanax treatment for three years before I met Dr. Spreen, who was helping me with some other related medical problems. I had hair loss, skin problems, nail-biting problems. I had aches all over my body, especially in my legs. Dr. Spreen got me on a vitamin regimen, which made me feel somewhat better.

"Then, last summer, Dr. Spreen put me on very low doses of thyroid and immediately—within two to three weeks—all the problems I just mentioned were gone. Now I had had thyroid checks three times during the whole time when I was being treated for infertility, and the blood tests had always come up negative. But I knew that in my family there were thyroid problems. There are at least six members of my family that I can think of who have thyroid disorders, but mine just never showed up on my tests. After taking these very low doses of thyroid, my skin problem cleared up, I stopped biting my nails, and my legs stopped aching. The mild depression I was still suffering from all of a sudden in August vanished. I felt great. I slept like a normal person again. I had energy. People started commenting on how I seemed to be like my old self again. It was like getting a new lease on life!

"I feel rather fed up with the original doctors I went to see. They treated me like I was an hysterical woman who needed to get a grip on things. I have never told them about my recovery using alternative methods because I don't think they'd be receptive to it. I did tell my therapist who has been very receptive to these new treatments and is most interested in

the thyroid treatments. But I'd say that the medical community is not open-minded about alternative treatments at all."

"Helen"

"I had hives, some kind of an allergic response, about five years ago and it progressed to the point where I had hives on my vocal chords. It was a pretty serious allergic reaction, for which I was first treated with antihistamines. Later, I was treated with prednisone. When small doses of prednisone given every other day didn't help, my doctor began increasing the dosage until I was taking 70 mg every day. After about six weeks I started declining physically from taking this tremendous dose. I gained about 50 pounds. I had conjunctivitis in both of my eyes. I had open sores. I was so weak I was almost bedridden. I did find another doctor who slowly weaned me off of the prednisone. But when it was all over, my immune system had been damaged. I had a lot of viral illnesses that are usually associated with chronic fatigue syndrome. I could scarcely get out of bed, and I couldn't lose all the weight I had gained. So I went from doctor to doctor. I was living in the Midwest at the time and many of these doctors said, 'Your metabolic system has been altered by prednisone. Too bad, but you will never lose that weight. And prednisone can damage the immune system. Too bad, but your immune system has been damaged.' No one could offer me any help at all.

"I first went to Dr. Atkins in New York and he was

a lot of help to me. It was through Dr. Atkins and his association with Dr. Huggins that I learned about dental amalgams, because when your immune system is depleted you are much more susceptible to any kind of toxins, including mercury leaching from mercury amalgam fillings. It was causing me a great deal of trouble and I did have those removed.

"Then I moved to California and I had heard, previous to my moving, about Dr. Slagle and her work with depression. In fact, I referred friends to her, friends I had made in California, and they had these miraculous cures from depression after two weeks of taking B-complex and amino acids. But I didn't think of going to her myself for quite awhile because I thought of her as someone who only treated depression. In fact, like many alternative physicians, she treats the whole person. She had worked with fatigue a lot, and she first tested me thoroughly and found that my thyroid and, in fact, my whole endocrine system, was not functioning properly— most likely as a result of prednisone. She picked up subtleties in the test that other doctors ignored. She has the philosophy that a body should be healthy and whole. She doesn't need gross parameters of unusual test results to say something is wrong here. So she was able to discover that I had a rather unusual problem in my thyroid and she was able to treat it.

"When I began seeing her I still had very limited energy. Even though Dr. Atkins had helped me lose weight so I looked normal, I still didn't feel normal. In one day, I could either go to the grocery store or go to a doctor's appointment. That was all I could

do. The remainder of the day I had to rest. I went to Dr. Slagle and after she began treating my thyroid I had a leap of improvement. I regained my energy. She also gave me amino acids, which heightened my mood. Even though I hadn't thought I was depressed—and I still don't think I was—generally the amino acids made me feel healthier. And while I don't have the energy of a lot of people around me, I can pretty much function normally, which is a miracle. It has been a five-year struggle and I'm finally living practically a normal life.

"Here's what I have learned from my experience. You simply cannot go to a traditional physician and carelessly allow that doctor to treat your symptoms with drugs. Traditional physicians tend not to look at the whole person, but to give drugs to ameliorate the symptoms, or to treat individual problems without regard to what that treatment does to the rest of the body. I learned to use tremendous caution when entrusting my body to someone. If you're going to trust your body to someone, you should know a lot about the physician. You should know whether the physician treats the whole person and sees you as more than an allergy or a gallbladder."

Nutritional and Environmental Influences on Mental States

18. Diet-Related Disorder

Thus far we've spoken about many specific mood and behavioral disorders, including eating disorders, that can be addressed through nutritional and holistic measures. We've also discussed a variety of specific treatable physical illnesses and imbalances that are often misdiagnosed as one or another type of resistant mental illness. In the following chapters, we zero in on a number of the environmental and nutritional elements, only referred to in earlier chapters, that can be key to our understanding and treatment of illnesses of the mind.

Dr. Robert Atkins describes the inaction of conventional physicians treating mental illness when it comes to identifying the root causes of any diet-related disorder. And in Dr. Atkins's opinion, depression and anxiety are both classifiable as diet-related disorders: "I have treated about 45,000 patients in my career. In just about every community around the country, psychiatrists are doing a sort of knee-jerk reaction to the problem of anxiety and depression. They never bother to ask, 'Why is my patient having a problem?' Instead, they immediately ask, 'What

145

is the name of the problem and what's its standard orthodox treatment?' They are bypassing the most important question of all: 'Why is my patient sick?'

"I would classify anxiety and depression under the general category of 'diet-related disorder.' By this I mean there is something in the diet that is actually contributing enough to this problem, so that if we correct the diet, the problem will disappear. The first question you have to ask is whether the symptoms change from hour to hour. Is the depression worse for an hour, and then it suddenly lifts? Does the anxiety change from hour to hour? That is the cardinal thing to look for because if the depression or anxiety are changeable, then they are almost definitely diet-related.

"What are the mechanisms of diet-related disorder? There are three major ones. The first—and the most important one— is blood-sugar instability. The old name was hypoglycemia, but that really doesn't describe it. It's the condition in which the blood sugar is capable of rapid escalations and rapid falls, so much so that the body is putting out other hormones—particularly adrenaline—to help regulate the blood sugar. Adrenaline is called forth when the blood sugar is on a free fall, which it usually does if something made it go up very fast, like a candy bar or a sugar and caffeine-laden cola drink. You can make your blood sugar go up very fast and if you have this problem, which, I would say, at least half the population has to some extent, then adrenaline is released and you get a panic attack. With the blood sugar instability, typically you get your reaction before a meal, if you haven't eaten, or if you have eaten sweets and then you haven't eaten anything else, which is the classical way to get it. That is really the basis of most anxiety states. Panic attacks can turn into an absolute phobia. You get a panic attack two or three times, and then become phobic in relation to whatever it was you were doing at the time you got your panic attack.

"The second mechanism is food allergies, which work a little differently. First you eat the offending food—which is often a grain, or milk, or sometimes some of the protein foods. Usually, the foods you are allergic to are whatever you eat most often, and since in our culture so many people eat bread with every meal, you have to suspect wheat. A lot of people drink milk with every meal, so dairy is a prime allergen. After eating foods you are allergic to over a long period of time, you may develop a leaky gut syndrome, and then you will develop the inability to handle the protein complexes that are characteristic of that food. So you get a reaction after you eat it.

"The third mechanism of this triumvirate," Dr. Atkins concludes, "is yeast, specifically candida albicans. The yeast itself is capable, through biochemical intermediaries, of making people a little 'flaky' right from the very beginning, but it also makes you more likely to have food intolerances, especially in people with sugar imbalances. Very often we will see people with all three of the above-mentioned conditions and they are going to a psychiatrist who is not trained to diagnose diet-related disorders. So even though you have psychiatric symptoms, you have a good chance of being incorrectly diagnosed because the doctor you are seeing does not specialize in diet-related disorders."

19. Food Allergies

There are two definitions of allergies today. The traditional, or classic, definition describes an immunological reaction, and, as Dr. Kendall Gerdes explains, "There are very good data suggesting that food allergies as traditionally defined are a fairly rare phenomenon—maybe three-tenths of one percent in children and even less in adults." Then there is the far more common phenomenon of food intolerance or hypersensitivity, which conventional doctors tend to know very little about. Again, Dr. Gerdes: "People read about food allergies in books they find in health food stores, but then they go to a traditional physician who thinks about allergies in a classic way. So he says, 'Well, this person is talking about something that is really rare.' But in fact, food intolerance or hypersensitivity is much more common. We have to be careful when we talk about allergies, to be sure we know whether we are speaking of the classical definition or the second, more common type.

"Many people do have significant symptoms related to foods, and these are not rare foods. They are not strawberries, or tomatoes, or peanuts that might be involved in the classic, more traditionally described immunological (IGE) food allergy reactions. They are instead hypersensitivities to the much more commonly eaten everyday foods, such as milk, wheat, and corn. These are the kinds of foods that can get to be problems.

"The immunoglobulin (IGE) E type reaction is really severe. That happens in the person who eats one peanut and has to be taken off to the emergency room. On the other hand, the kind of food sensitivity I am talking about occurs in people who eat fairly large amounts of a particular food, and many times they can't see the cause-and-effect relationship because they are eating that food all the time.

"The first people to do research in the area of food intolerance did so 40 to 50 years ago," Dr. Gerdes continues. "A physician named Herbert Rinkel was the first one to observe that a food a person ate all the time might be causing symptoms, but you couldn't see the relationship. If you took the person off that food for a week and then gave it to them, then you might get a sharp and clear reaction. He called this 'masked food allergy.'

"Dr. Theron Randolph enlarged the concept. He observed that not only did people use these foods often, but they used the foods as if they were addicted to them. They didn't merely have wheat for breakfast, they craved wheat. They loved wheat. They might have it six times a day. They might even, if they had trouble sleeping, eat wheat in the middle of the night to help them get back to sleep. And he found that when people were using certain foods in this kind of pattern, they temporarily felt better after eating the food. By using the same principles that Dr. Rinkel had used, Dr. Randolph would take the person off the food for a week and then challenge them. In that way, many times he could see the reaction that the patient themselves could not see. The

149

critical variable was, once he began to look for the foods that people were addicted to, he found he had a much better basis from which to determine the foods to which people were allergic.

"A person might have a wide array of emotional and mental reactions. He or she might be irritable, depressed, or anxious because of foods that they are eating or because of chemicals in their environment such as perfumes or formaldehyde in particle board or furniture. Research is only beginning to understand how this process works. Dr. Iris Bell, a professor of psychiatry at the University of Arizona, is very interested in this topic and has been exploring it more than anyone else. She is finding that food and chemical sensitivities probably play into the endorphin system—the same system that produces a runner's high. The endorphin system is used as a way for the brain to give a feeling of comfort. For instance, when an infant is crying or upset, the mother gives him some breast milk, and the sugar and fat in the milk probably trigger the endorphin system so that the baby then can go to sleep. That same system can be activated under some circumstances by children and adults in order to make themselves feel good. As a consequence, people find themselves having to use a particular food or a group of foods to make themselves feel better. That is part of the basis of food addiction.

"The simplest approach to use in order to figure out what foods you are sensitive to is to look for the foods that you are using a lot, if you are someone whose symptoms seem to fluctuate over the course of an hour, a day, or a week. This is the same approach that most of the physicians in the Academy of Environmental Medicine use, among others.

"Here's a hypothetical 35-year-old woman. (I say a woman because women go to doctors more frequently than men do, for whatever the reason. Whether this is because men are being more stoic and not coming in, or whether women are more vulnerable, we don't really know.) It would not be uncommon to find a woman who has a fair amount of fatigue, with a low-grade depression that sometimes gets to the point where she almost can't cope with things. When that occurs, and it is a variable type of thing, I will look for the two, or five, or ten foods that she is using a lot and suggest that she take them out of her diet for a week. Then, at the end of that week, many times she will find that she is not so tired and doesn't have that low-grade depression; she has more motivation to do things. Then I get more specific and test one food at a time. I ask her to have a big meal of each of those foods that she has been avoiding. Many times we can find out which food or foods have been causing the low-grade depression and her other symptoms. Though this is a generic example," Dr. Gerdes concludes, "cases just like it are fairly common."

Dr. Abram Hoffer offers another case study: "I treated a young man who was both schizophrenic and alcoholic. He had been working on his Ph.D. when he became so ill that he could not continue. Eventually he came under my care. It turned out that he didn't respond too well to my program—the vitamins and the other things that I was doing—and finally I discovered from his mother, not from him, that he consumed 12 ounces of tomato juice every morning, and had since he was a child. That was one of his basic breakfast foods. And it turned out that he had a tomato allergy. Then his mother told me that she too had been allergic to tomatoes, but she hadn't touched them for at least 60 years.

"When I put the young man on a tomato-free diet, and explained to him why, his depression and his schizophrenia vanished and he became normal. He was my second case in which a food allergy was a major factor in determining the illness of a person. It can be any one food or often a combination of foods—two or even three foods—that people have to learn to avoid, and their mental condition will then improve dramatically."

20. Heavy Metal Toxicity

Dr. Richard Kunin emphasizes the importance of hair tests, as opposed to the blood tests which are performed more commonly, in the prevention of heavy metal poisoning. To start off, Dr. Kunin offers a personal account of heavy metal toxicity from his own family's experience: "A beautiful son was born to me in October 1971. In about June of 1972, he had enough hair for a hair test and I did one, and found that he had roughly 80 parts per million of lead in his hair. He should have had zero. Eighty parts per million is a toxic load and could only be coming from something he was eating. It was not something that we were putting on his hair; we certainly didn't use hair sprays or dyes. So I knew that my son, before he was a year old, was already poisoned. My heart fell. I almost fainted with grief. We checked things out and found that a toy that had been given as a gift was tainted with six percent lead in the paint—that's 6,000 parts per million. If we hadn't done a hair test, he would have continued to have been poisoned and would have been mentally retarded.

"Lead poisoning has, first, a bad effect on the brain. The second bad effect is that you get bowel problems and colic. The third thing is you lose your coordination because the hands and feet are weak. Then the immune system is weakened. In other words, you are just not the person you could have been.

"I once had an 18-year-old patient, a beautiful woman, who came to see me who was depressed. She graduated from college with a C average and was disappointed in herself. She had been raised on vitamins and an Adelle Davis diet by a very caring mother. But they had lived overseas, where they had bought native pottery, and as a baby she was already lead-poisoned. I know this because I did a hair analysis of the child's hair samples that her mother had saved at various ages. At one and a half, her hair was 180 parts per million of lead. At five, it was down to 80. At age 12 it was down to practically nothing, and at age 18 we couldn't find it. As she grew, this load of lead that she had picked up as a baby was being absorbed into her tissues and being diluted. But it left behind its damage on her. Her teachers would write on her report card, 'Jennifer could have done so much better if she had really tried.' The teachers couldn't understand it. The girl had an attention deficit based on an early-life toxicity that went undiagnosed because nobody looked.

"In an enlightened society, all children should be tested for lead. But their hair and not their blood should be tested. The government is spending millions of dollars to test children by taking a blood sample for lead, which is absolutely ridiculous. Lead will be filtered out of the blood in a week. If you are exposed to lead this week, by next week it will be gone, but it will remain in your hair for six months. When a hair test is done once a year, you are going to find lead contamination if it is present.

"Hair analysis, for a reasonable price, gives you 30 or more real facts about the levels of mercury, arsenic, cadmium, lead, nickel, aluminum, and fluoride that have built up in your body. Everyone should know what toxic substances and physiologic minerals—chromium, selenium, boron—they're accumulating or are deficient in. We have very few tools that give us this kind of perspective," Dr. Kunin concludes. "The contamination level can be minute and still show up on the test, whose accuracy is quite high."

Dr. Christopher Calapai details some of the sources of our exposure to heavy metal contamination, and how the problem can be so damaging to our mental and physical health: "We are exposed to metals from a wide variety of places. They are in our drinking water, in some of our foods, even in our work environment where we breathe in certain toxins. Lead, for example, can come into the body through exposure to metals in paints. We get cadmium from our food, air, and water; mercury from dental fillings and shellfish; and aluminum and excess iron from pots and pans. Many of the metals that are brought into the body are toxic to the brain and to central nervous system tissue. They interfere with normal metabolism by disrupting enzyme systems.

"Here is how the textbook *Aluminum and Alzheimer's Disease: An Update* presents the relationship between aluminum and mercury poisoning and disease: 'There have been reports of increased aluminum in the bulk of brain tissue in Alzheimer's patients and more recently associations of aluminum with neurofibrillary tangles and neuritic plaques. Aluminum has also been associated with neurofibrillary degeneration in patients with amyotrophic lateral sclerosis and Parkinsonism type dementia. Mercury is released during the placement and removal of amalgams. Areas of concern with regard to mercury exposure include kidney dysfunction, neurotoxicity, reduced immune function, hypersensitivity reactions, birth defects and overall changes in general health.'

"The *Food Additives Handbook* reports that lead, cadmium, and arsenic are put into animal feed, as are other heavy metals. They are probably placed there intentionally to remove germs. In addition, aluminum is found in baking powder, table salt, and vanilla powder. It's used as an emulsifier, and as an anti-caking agent," Dr. Calapai adds.

Testing and treatment protocols for heavy metal poisoning should be holistic and should take into consideration recent refinements in treatment. As Dr. Calapai explains, "When testing for heavy metal toxicity, you want to take the entire patient into consideration. Are they having any symptoms that can be related to an exposure to heavy metals? Have they had numerous dental procedures? Do they have decreased memory? Have there been changes in their behavior or mood?

"Before treating the condition, we perform a blood test to check vitamin and mineral levels, we examine the person's diet, consider what they do for work, where they work, and what they're exposed to at work, as well as in their home environment. We also do a 24-hour urine test with an intravenous chelation procedure, and test for creatinine clearance (kidney function), as well as testing for heavy metals.

"The latest and best treatment of heavy metal toxicity is a combination of oral vitamins and minerals to maximize immune function, exercise, and intravenous EDTA chelation therapy to remove the metals. Vitamin C is also beneficial. Some people use intravenous vitamin C and alternate that with chelation.

"The vitamins and minerals that we recommend are based upon the individual's particular needs. We check to see if the patient is deficient in different nutrients or if they're not absorbing certain nutrients present in their diet. The ranges are individually different and depend on the result of the physical exam."

Dr. Calapai also discusses chelation therapy, an important modality to treat heavy metal poisoning, as well as certain other illnesses, including heart disease in some cases: "Chelation therapy is a treatment that has been around for many years. It involves using an intravenous application or induction of a protein substance that helps to bind heavy metals, to drag them out and throw them out of the body through the urine. The treatment takes about three hours to perform. It also has been shown to produce significant changes in plaque deposition in the lining of blood vessels, so it can help to open up and improve blood circulation in the body. You can detect how well the metals are being removed by means of a repeat 24-hour urine test. Chelation therapy for people who have heavy metal toxicity may be done once or twice a week for 15 weeks," Dr. Calapai concludes.

Holistic practitioners don't always scorn conventional sources of information. Instead, they seek to find ways in which their training in traditional Western medicine and their, usually more recent, interest in holistic approaches, can complement one another. On the subject of heavy metal poisoning, Dr. Alfred Zamm refers us to a medical school textbook: "The standard conservative medical school textbook, *The Textbook of Pharmacology*, by Goodman and Gilman, contains the following passage about mercury, 'Doctors very rarely make the diagnosis of mercury poisoning because the symptoms are so varied. It comes in many disguises.'

"To paraphrase the text," Zamm continues, "Mercury poisoning is like a ghost. You don't know it's there. It comes and goes, wearing masks. Some years ago, I wrote an article called

157

'The Removal of Dental Mercury—Often an Effective Treatment for the Very Sensitive Patient,' and I listed as many as 50 symptoms associated with mercury poisoning. The top three of the 50 were fatigue, inappropriate coldness, and sugar intolerance. These patients will crave sugar and eat sweet things, and may or may not know that they will get sick. They may eat sweets on Monday and get sick on Tuesday. They may have all sorts of bizarre symptoms—muscle aches and pains, fatigue, headaches, personality changes. Remember, you don't have to have all of the symptoms to have mercury poisoning. You can have one, and it may come and go."

Here are some other common symptoms of mercury poisoning, according to Dr. Zamm: headaches, difficulty concentrating, difficulty with reading comprehension, forgetfulness, depression, and skin changes. "It is very difficult," he adds, "to prove mercury poisoning, except after the fact when the mercury is out and the patient feels better. Now taking a whole group of fillings out is not a minor matter. So I have devised some tests that people can do themselves in order to assess whether or not it is worth proceeding in this direction.

"First of all," Zamm explains, "if you crave sugar and sugar makes you sick, and you are already suspicious about that, then take this test. First, try taking selenium, which is a mineral that binds with mercury, cadmium, and arsenic. If you feel better after taking selenium, it is a clue, not a diagnosis. About 20 years ago, when I started to investigate selenium, I realized that there was a paradox. Some people got better right away, some people took about three months, and some people got worse. I finally figured out that the patients who got worse were those who were most sensitive. They were the ones who were really sick—the ones who needed it the most but because of a peculiar intolerance

158

to everything, including the things they needed, couldn't deal with the selenium. To overcome this, I had the very sensitive patients dilute chemically pure selenium down to very small dilutions. By starting with very small dilutions and gradually building up the dosage over a period of three months, these very sick patients started to get better."

Dr. Zamm's experience with selenium is a powerful reminder, supported in the literature, of the importance of this issue: "Aside from tying up these toxic substances—mercury, cadmium, and arsenic—selenium is also protective against cancer. A study was done by a man named Schroeder at Dartmouth. He investigated 50 cities in the United States, found their cancer rates, and rated them from highest to lowest. Then he also found out the selenium content of their water and lined them up. The cities with the highest selenium had the lowest cancer rate, and vice versa. Later on, this correlation turned out to be causally connected.

"Selenium does provide protection against cancer—probably due to its tying up of toxic metals like cadmium, arsenic, and mercury. Moreover, selenium is an atom that fits into a molecule called glutathionperoxidase, which helps to destroy dangerous, foreign chemicals that just don't belong in our bodies, such as petrochemicals, floor wax, and insecticides. So when you take selenium, you're not only knocking out mercury, cadmium, and arsenic, you are also helping to produce more glutathionperoxidase, which protects you from environmental contaminants. So if you feel better, it is not an absolute diagnosis of mercury poisoning.

"Within pyruvate dehydrogenase complex, there are three enzymes. The first one uses thiamine, vitamin B_1. If you are tired all the time, and you take 25 mg of thiamine once or twice a day, which is a low dose, and you notice you feel better, that is another clue you might have mercury poisoning. Now you have the selenium and the thiamine clue.

"The last thing is zinc. If you look at the periodic table that shows how the elements are arranged, you'll notice that there is a column containing zinc, cadmium, and mercury, in order from top to bottom. If you have too much cadmium and mercury in the body, they will replace zinc in the enzymes. Now our bodies have 50 to 75 enzymes with zinc in them. So if you have mercury knocking out your zinc, then you know why it is poisoning you. It is inactivating enzymes by knocking out the zinc, which is supposed to be there, and replacing it with mercury which doesn't work. This is cellular poisoning. You are not burning sugar, which is why you are cold and tired, and that's why you are sugar-intolerant.

"Why do some people who have mercury in their bodies not get sick? In a speech I gave at the FDA in March 1991, I explained the reason. We are all different; some of us are small, some tall. It's the same thing with enzymes. We are genetically polymorphic, meaning that some people have a lot of enzymes that work very well and some people have less and what they have doesn't work very well. Some of us who have mercury in our bodies are able to deal with it, while others are not able to deal with it. Those who are just getting by, who were born with a slight deficiency, will just get through. But if, at age 12 or 13, people are poisoned by having mercury fillings put in their mouths, those who have strong enzyme systems may not notice much, but those who are less strong start to manifest symptoms, although usually not right away. After a few months, a child can't concentrate at school. Maybe he or she develops allergies, and nobody connects it with the filling that was put in six months earlier.

"I have seen patients with a single filling who experience problems. One woman, a Russian emigrant who had no fillings, at age 20 got a single filling. She came to me at 22 with a shopping bag full of medicine. She didn't know what was wrong with her. She couldn't think. She was nauseated and sick all the time. When I asked her when it all started, she said it had been two years ago. I looked into her mouth, and saw the single filling, and asked her when she had gotten it. She said it had been put in two years ago. I asked which had come first, the filling or the illness. And she said, 'Oh my God. It was three months after the filling was put in that I got sick.' She was a very skeptical woman who didn't trust American medicine or anything. I told her she had to have it taken out. She was so desperate that she said, 'I don't believe a word you are saying but I'm going to have it taken out because I'm afraid that I will die if I don't.'

"She had the filling removed. In 17 days, she was able to start eating some foods that she couldn't eat before. It took about three months before she saw some substantial results and she came back and said to me, 'I believe it.' Now that was a problem caused by a single filling.

"I have one patient, a young child, who had a filling the size of a pinhead and I didn't see it because it was in the back. You'd need a special dental mirror. And I said to the mother, 'I don't understand this case. This child can't tolerate sugar, he is hyperkinetic.' (Hyperkinesis, or hyperactivity, is one of the symptoms of mercury poisoning.) I said, 'This has to be a case of mercury poisoning. This child was perfectly well until he was seven. But I don't see any fillings.' She said, 'Doctor, there is a filling there.' So I got a dental mirror from a colleague of mine and looked. Sure enough, there was a filling the size of a pinhead. I couldn't believe it. I had the filling removed, and within three months the child was substantially improved. This child was genetically polymorphic in the sense that he had a very inefficient oxidation process.

"When you talk about genetically polymorphic individuals who are sensitive, such as the Russian emigrant woman, they are going to have many of the symptoms that I have mentioned, including depressions, anxiety, and sleep disturbances. If you are not oxidizing, if you are not burning sugar, you are energy-deficient and you are going to be deficient in many other organ functions. Mercury poisoning from dental fillings is so elusive because it is in effect sabotaging the engine of their lives. Each organ will express itself in its own dysfunction. That is why muscle aches and depression and all those things go together. But some organs are a little stronger than others so they won't manifest symptoms.

"If a patient comes in and says, 'I'm depressed,' one of the causes may be mercury poisoning. I once gave a lecture to a group of graduate students in psychology because the chairman of the department, who was my patient, was so impressed with the fact that you could get the patient better physically and affect the mental illness. The title of the lecture was 'How I Would Like to Be Treated if I Were a Patient.'

"I said, in short: 'First, we have to make sure the patient is physically healthy. Let the patient be investigated by a good internist who gives a thorough physical examination, assuming nothing. Next, we want to make sure that the person doesn't have allergies. Third, we ascertain whether or not the person has biochemical disruptions, from exposure to toxic elements, including mercury. Only after we've done steps one, two, and three, can we go to step four, which is to recommend going to speak to a psychologist.'

"In the case of mercury poisoning, there may be enough oxygen available, but the person's body can't burn it because the burning mechanism has shut down. In every case of depression, physical deficiencies and toxic poisoning should be considered first, before resorting to therapy and psychotropic medications such as antidepressants. I have seen hundreds of these cases respond to diagnosis and treatment of the underlying physical cause.

"How is it possible that, in the 1990s, dentists are continuing to put a toxic substance in our mouths? We need some historical perspective on the issue. In 1826, a Parisian named Taveau discovered that if you took silver coins and filed them into dust and mixed it with mercury, and then squeezed the mercury out, this putty would harden quickly. Then you could take this putty-like material, push it into a cavity in someone's mouth, and it would harden like concrete. Other people realized that this wasn't such a good idea and there were arguments back and forth. Then, in 1833 in New York, two brothers went into the business of doing this process on a mass scale. It's a cheap filling. You don't have to be a good dentist to make a mercury filling.

"The so-called silver amalgam filling is a lie. This 'silver' filling is only 30 percent silver, but it is 50 percent mercury and 20 percent various other metals that can produce hardness. They call it a silver filling when the major ingredient is mercury. So I refer to it as a mercury filling.

"To give you some perspective on just how long ago 1826 was, in terms of the degree of ignorance that was then prevalent, consider that in 1860, 35 years later, a man in Vienna said to doctors, 'If you don't wash your hands before you examine pregnant women, you are going to spread disease.' And this man was thrown out of the medical society because he was impugning the reputation of physicians. They didn't know about germs in those days. It was not until 1875 that Louis Pasteur and others proved that germs were a major cause of disease. And yet dental technology invented back in the medical Dark Ages is what we are still using today, nearly 175 years later.

"How can mercury fillings still be considered to be safe? The answer: If you did it before, it's okay to do it again. For example, lead pipes were the standard for years, so they are still okay now. Luckily, we have finally gotten around to seeing that lead pipes weren't really safe, that the lead leaching into the water causes brain damage. So we've stopped using lead in pipes. We still have tobacco from when the colonists smoked it with the Indians hundreds of years ago. You still can't convince some people that it's not healthy to smoke. We continue to sell tobacco and other poisonous substances out of habit and the profit motive.

"The same is true with mercury fillings. There is no proof that they are safe. Now, if you went out to buy a can of soup in the supermarket, it would be strange to have the clerk behind the counter say to you, 'I'd like you to prove the safety of this can.' You would say, 'What are you talking about? I'm purchasing the can. The fact that you are selling it implies that you are saying that it's safe.' But the clerk says, 'Not when it comes to soup. When it comes to soup, it is the responsibility of the purchaser to prove that it is safe or not safe. We as the sellers don't have to do anything.' That's the situation we're in with mercury fillings. No one has ever proved that mercury fillings are safe in human beings. They should prove it. But instead, the dental industry has turned it around and said, 'No, you have to prove it is unsafe.' They say it is safe but they haven't proven it."

Dr. Zamm concludes: "We are continuing to use a 175-year-old anachronistic mixture of crude coin filings mixed with mercury. And we are walking around with this mixture in our teeth without any proof of safety. Charlemagne said, 'If the populace knew with what idiocy they were ruled, they would revolt.' That goes for some of the things that they do in dentistry, too."

Dr. Ray Wunderlich offers another example of heavy metal toxicity: "A 30-year-old worker from an orange juice plant in Florida, who was a chemist and had been working there for about three years, came to me because she was depressed, irritable, and anxious; she felt like her brain was in a fog. I did a chemical analysis of this patient: I looked at her blood—her red cells and her plasma—her urine, and her hair. The results showed that she had excesses of five toxic metals: arsenic, cadmium, lead, aluminum, and copper. Now, she had an occupational exposure to heavy metals. Many systems had gone off in the body of this relatively young woman. When she was treated for heavy metal toxicity, she progressively improved and got well. Her case is a very dramatic example of mental dysfunction and emotional problems that cleared up with the elimination of toxins.

"In the U.S.," Dr. Wunderlich continues, "there's a lot of background exposure to heavy metals. Think about all of the auto tires on the road that are spinning off cadmium in their wheels as they wear down, all the 50,000 chemicals in the environment that weren't there 50 years ago. We are all being exposed to toxins. Dr. Davis from England has shown that these gradually and insidiously accumulate in our systems with every decade that we live. So we have to face the strong likelihood that this toxic build-up is interfering with our enzyme function."

21. Chemicals and Other Environmental Factors Contributing to Mental Conditions

The risk of being exposed to chemicals such as pesticides in our environment is constantly increasing. A variety of common illnesses, including certain types of depression, can be traced to chemical and environmental toxicity as their root cause. Dr. Richard Kunin offers two case histories where exposure to chemicals and other environmental factors were decisive, and where proper diagnosis by a holistic practitioner led to a successful treatment outcome. "Once at a dinner party I met a woman and it turned out that the party was at the home of her psychoanalyst who was a transactional therapist, a psychiatrist, and also an M.D. And she was a victim of a depression that would come and go. The conversation turned to what kind of therapy a doctor like myself—an orthomolecular doctor and a nutrition physician—would use. She decided to come in for a consultation to explain her depressions. In the first two months, as I went through phase one with her, which was the nutrition analysis stage, nothing came of it.

"There was almost a 100-percent probability that we were going to find something chemical because the psychological inputs just didn't explain her depressions. So we went back over the whole case and hit upon something she had forgotten to tell me the first time around, which was that after she had had her third child by Cesarean, she hadn't been able to breathe for a day. Probing further, we found that the anesthesia she was administered was accompanied by a paralysis of her respiratory muscles. It's a short-term muscle relaxant that blocks the neural muscular junction and the transmitter and you are supposed to recover in a matter of minutes. She recovered in a day. If they had not had an automatic pressure respirator there she would have died.

"She has a potentially fatal disorder. When she was measured they found that her detoxifying enzyme, called cholinesterase, which is supposed to get rid of a chemical like this, was abnormally low on a genetic basis. Now she knew about this but nobody explained to her that it put her at risk for environmental exposure to pesticides that would damage this enzyme further. The common phosphate pesticides were life-threatening to this woman. Nobody told her. Now it turns out that she is a well-to-do woman who could afford to have an exterminator come in and spray her kitchen every month or two. And she would be disabled. The pesticide sprays are supposed to last about a week but it takes about two to three weeks to recover for an ordinary exposure and with her low cholinesterase she would be out for a month.

"She would feel depressed, weak, and shaky. She would have

intestinal bloat. She would wheeze a little. She would sleep poorly, have strange dreams. Her saliva would be a little thin. In general, her autonomic nervous system was a wreck.

"When she would visit her family up in Napa Valley, California, which is full of vineyards that are sprayed, everyone else would be playing tennis, and she would be in bed with the covers over her head. Everyone thought that she was neurotic. Nobody measured her cholinesterase until I heard the story, checked, and, sure enough, found she had a genetic deficiency.

"In my own practice, I have come upon four cases like this, about one every two years. But in addition to these four, there have been well over 60 people I've seen in the past six or seven years who don't have the advanced or severe form, but have a milder form of environmental susceptibility. One of these was a nurse who was in the hospital on the psychiatric ward for depression. Although her condition was improving at the hospital, she knew that this wasn't the answer. She wasn't even on medication. Just being in the ward, she was getting better, which already tells us something. She wasn't at home. She was in a new environment, and so the suspicion of environmental factors having an impact goes up.

"This is an important point. If you go on a vacation and feel better, it doesn't necessarily mean that you needed a vacation. Maybe you needed to be out of your home territory where there are environmental factors that make you sick. Now in my practice I always measure cholinesterase levels. This nurse's cholinesterase were also below the normal limit. It turned out that whenever she was visiting her home territory, which was rural, she would be aware that they were spraying by airplane. From a mile away this woman would pick up drifts and her immune system was responding to the solvents and detergents that are used to disperse the sprays over a wide area. But when we measured her cholinesterase, we found that it fluctuated. When it went down—meaning it was inactivated by pesticide exposure—then she would have more symptoms, particularly depressions. When she would recover and be at her high level—meaning she was not impaired—she would feel perfectly healthy and normal and was a vivacious, dynamic person.

"I call this the 'pesticide neurosis.' It's not rare and it's a very significant factor, because people are reacting to common, so-called 'safe' pesticides. These are the same pesticides that California sprayed all over the city of Los Angeles, where there were people who were having all kinds of symptoms, especially when they would spray in two adjacent areas consecutively. If you lived in the cusp between two areas, you got a double dose.

"These are the most common pesticide problems that show up as everyday nerve problems. If you eat out in restaurants, they are sprayed every few weeks, and chances are you are going to pick up some of the leftovers of some of these commercial pesticides. They are careful and they do it well, but accidents do happen. If you are having symptoms of environmental susceptibility, you have got to include this in your thinking. Doctors should be including it in their testing."

Dr. Kunin continues: "Judging from the 30 or 40 cases of environmental toxicity that I could refer to from my own clinical experience, it is fairly common for a patient to have a family history. You'll find out that cousin Joe had it or you'll hear that there was a suicide in the family. In fact this may have been the case with the nurse I've been describing. She came to see me looking for nutrition-related answers, and we found instead a toxin-related answer for her. She had a cousin who lived in the San Mateo area, south of San Francisco. When we had the Med

Fly scare back in 1983, after the area where her cousin lived was sprayed, he went into a terrible depression and committed suicide. Of course, I can't prove that the depression was brought on by a toxic reaction to the spraying. I didn't get a blood level on him. But when you have one person with a family history of an enzyme weakness and another person with related genes who goes into a deep depression after having been exposed to a bad environmental onslaught, you have to at least consider that the two events are causally related.

"These kinds of stories are a wake-up call. Even at this late stage, while we assume everyone is so aware and concerned about pesticides, that is not the case. The government agencies and the higher-ups in the medical political structure are not even half-aware, and the actual interventions that we've seen to date are only partial. As for members of the medical profession generally, they do not really take environmental toxicity seriously. They see it as very rare and therefore they don't include hair analysis as part of a routine medical checkup. In fact, doctors have been told *not* to test for toxins, even though these tests are the best way to screen for poisonous metals as well as to identify how much of various minerals a person is accumulating in the tissues of his or her body," Dr. Kunin concludes.

Dr. Michael Schachter looks for clues in his patients' behavioral habits. Here is one case of a patient with pronounced chemical sensitivities, from his clinical practice: "One woman, whom I have been treating for some time now, becomes very depressed and even has auditory hallucinations when exposed to formaldehyde in department stores. Recently, she was able to improve her condition by using a detoxification program in which she took sauna baths and certain nutrients, such as niacin and vitamin C. It took several weeks of a couple of hours a day of low heat saunas to remove some of the toxic chemicals that were in the fat stores of her body. One possibly relevant factor in her history was that as an adolescent she had engaged in substance abuse, including both marijuana and hallucinogenic drugs like LSD. Though she has improved considerably, she continues to be sensitive to chemicals."

"Betty:" A Personal Account of Environmental Toxicity

"Back in 1991, I was injured on the job from some paint fumes and my whole life changed. I developed serious food allergies and sensitivities to everything in my environment. I became allergic to everything in my own home, I reacted to plastics of all kinds, and I couldn't breathe outdoor air. When I couldn't go out, all the air inside my own home had to be filtered especially for me and I had to wear charcoal face masks to breathe. I was literally a captive in my own home for the first year. Also, I began to experience depressions, mood swings, and a lot of confusion and memory loss. I would go into one room and forget why I was there. I know a lot of people have that complaint from time to time, but I had it consistently throughout the day. I would lose my memory about what I was doing while I was doing it. I couldn't go out in the car and drive myself to the store because I wouldn't be able to find my way. I lost the ability to read normally. Still now, two years later, I have to read things over and over in order to retain the material. I still have that deficit. I have trouble dealing with numbers.

"Unfortunately, because my chemical exposure

happened to me on the job, I became a workers' compensation patient. This meant that I was very often sent to doctors who were unwilling to believe that there was something wrong with me or who didn't understand what the syndrome was all about. So for months at a time, because of their diagnoses, I would go without any treatment at all and I would just get worse. This period of being a captive in my own home, with other members of my family doing all my usual daily activities, such as shopping, lasted about a year.

"Luckily I found several doctors who were able to diagnose and treat me with various methods. Dr. Wunderlich was one of the first of these doctors and he helped me quite a bit. He administered vitamin C drips, a vitamin supplement program, and allergy treatments, because every allergy that you can think of was triggered in my body. I had a total allergy syndrome. I had become allergic to everything that I breathed in and everything that I put on my skin. To this day, I cannot use any kind of lotions, cosmetics, fragrances, or hair sprays, and I doubt that I ever will be able to use them.

"Very slowly I began to get better. I still have frequent setbacks because of chemical exposures. I can't tolerate anything like gasoline fumes, new plastics, or any kind of new materials in a building. I have very restricted access to public places because of fragrances that are often used in offices, stores, or public restrooms, and because of cleaning solutions and sprays used in public places. So now, after two years, I am still slowly making progress. But from everything that I have learned, I have

several more years ahead of me before I can bring my immune system back to where it should be.

"I like people and I have always, all of my life, been around people. One of my greatest frustrations has been that now I find I have to dodge people because of the cosmetics, perfumes, and sprays that they use. A big part of my life is spent dodging people in order to protect myself from these things. They set off severe migraine attacks that can put me into bed for two and three days at a time.

"I was forced into changing my lifestyle. I had to change my way of eating, and my way of living. I had to change a lot of the products that I use in my home to nontoxic products, like baking soda and vinegar solutions. Now, that is all I use in my home. I've gone to a semi-vegetarian diet. Most of my vegetables are organic. I eat very little meat, and no flavorings. I have to be on a completely yeast-free and sugar-free diet. It is an extremely restricted diet. But I have gotten used to it and I realize now that it's an extremely healthy diet. It's a natural diet, the type of diet that people probably ate 50 or 60 years ago.

"My experience with various doctors has made me see the need for more physician awareness. So many physicians saw me as a neurotic middle-aged woman because of the symptoms that I had. The symptoms that go with environmental illness are numerous and have to be taken seriously by the medical profession. It is not all in our heads."

Behavioral, Affective, and Mental Disorders in Children

22. *Aggression*

Often, those most susceptible to environmental illnesses, and to misdiagnoses by conventionally trained physicians, are also those who are least able to protect themselves from the dangers these problems pose. Our children live in environments we create for them, and they either benefit by or suffer from the changes we make in those environments. A range of behavioral, affective, and mental disorders affects children primarily. They are discussed in the following chapters.

In many cases, the culprit is found to be environmental toxins of one type or another. Dr. Harold Buttram points out that while most of our knowledge of the effect of environmental toxins comes from reports of occupational exposure in adults, there is no doubt that developing children are at even greater risk for developing environmental toxin-related illnesses. "It is a known fact that pesticides are toxic to the nervous system. Most of our knowledge in this area comes from studies of occupational exposures in adults. What is not known—and all the texts say this—is how toxic are the continual low-dose exposures that are commonly incurred from the environment, and especially, how toxic they are to children. The evidence suggests that there is sufficient toxicity, from residual pesticides in foods, air, and water, and in homes and yards, to cause neurotoxic damage—particularly to children or to the fetus during pregnancy.

"All the scientific literature emphasizes that the fetus and young children are far more vulnerable to toxic chemicals than adults are," Dr. Buttram adds. "And yet the government standards for limitations of pesticides are set by adult standards, which do not take into account the heightened susceptibility of children.

"In order to assess the damage caused by pesticides and other toxic chemicals to the nervous and immune systems in children, every educated person should read a government publication entitled *Neurotoxicity: Identifying and Controlling Poisons of the Nervous System*. It points out that behavioral problems are one of the earliest signs of chemical toxicity, which is what we are seeing in children today. In fact, researchers in the field of chemical toxicity are extremely concerned about the impact of environmental chemicals on children."

As Dr. Doris Rapp explains, aggression, an important issue for some children, often has an environmental root cause. "Aggression can be due to dust, pollen, molds, foods, and chemicals. Any of these things can turn an absolute angel into a tyrant in seconds. A frequent clue to an allergic reaction is that affected children develop red earlobes, wiggly legs, red cheeks, a red nose, and sometimes a spacey look in the eyes. At times these children can be very nasty and aggressive, with a frightening demonic look in their eyes. They throw out their lower lip and their eyes are half-shut and they look as if they are going to kill you. I've seen this in three-year-old children who eat the wrong food, or if we just take one drop of an allergy extract containing a substance to which they are sensitive and prick their arm with it.

"We have videotapes documenting what we're talking about. However, insurance companies are very reluctant to pay for this kind of medical care, even though many times specialists in environmental medicine can see patients and relieve symptoms that haven't been helped by all the other medical specialists. They pay for medical care that does not help and don't pay for care that does help. We must ask why. Insurance companies say environmental medicine is experimental and anecdotal. If we take two hours taking a history and do extensive patient or parent teaching to show them how to figure out answers so they can finally detect what's causing the problem, on a long-term basis, it is time well spent. That individual stands a chance of remaining well and not needing drugs or hospitalization once the true cause has been identified and eliminated. Insurance companies should be delighted because, in the long run, this approach saves an enormous amount of their money, as well as preserving the well-being and preventing the heartache for so many patients and family members.

"Insurance companies are reluctant to pay the environmental specialist, but will very quickly pay the hospital. Each day in the hospital can cost $1000. The total cost for environmental treatment of a serious condition would be much less than a week in the hospital.

"I have seen a number of children who have been so difficult in school that they have been singled out by school officials. First, all the usual quieting drugs were tried, and when nothing helped, they were told that they would have to be institutionalized. We have videotapes showing that these same children can be turned around. They act great, until we give them a particular food to eat or skin test them with one drop of an allergy extract solution containing the item that bothers them. Within minutes, they are absolutely uncontrollable. Four people have to hold them down. They are spitting, hitting, kicking, and then we give them the right one drop, the correct dilution of that same substance that caused the problem, and they are right back to normal. This newer, more precise, allergy detection is called provocation/neutralization allergy testing. No, we can't explain why this happens. The body is smarter than the doctors.

"I have a number of patients who were going to be institutionalized and who did not need to be. I have seen many other children who were put in classes for the learning disabled because they've been classified as learning disabled or as having conceptual understanding problems or perceptual disorders of various sorts. Many times they fall between the cracks. The school doesn't know how to classify them, if, for example, they display 'autistic-like' behavior. Some (although certainly not all) of these children have responded beautifully to allergy care. Their grades go up significantly. One child's IQ changed from 57 to 125 in a period of 19 months. Some of the children have been returned to be in the classroom with their peers. Many of them can switch from home teaching to school if the parent can pay to have an air purifier put in the classroom," Dr. Rapp concludes.

"Brittany:" A Personal Account of Aggression

"I am Brittany's mother. Just after she was born, when she was about three weeks old, she started having recurring ear infections. She was always going on antibiotics—literally every two weeks— until she was about two years old. At that time a friend introduced us to an allergist in Massachusetts,

who put her through allergy testing and treatment. We changed our daughter's diet after finding that there were certain foods to which she was severely allergic, such as chicken, sugar, and dairy.

"After a year of allergy therapy, she is doing much better. She is a relatively calm child; she can play nicely by herself and has a very good temperament. She is one of these kids that, if you have to give her an injection, she'll just sit there and maybe giggle. But when she has sugar or chicken, she turns into a little animal. She becomes extremely cranky, gets almost violent. She will want to hit you; she will cling to me and to her father.

"We didn't understand what was happening until we started to see a pattern. When we found out she was allergic to these things, we started to understand that eating these foods was what caused the tantrum-like behavior. Also, her infections completely stopped during the treatment. When she went off of the allergy treatments for a little while, because our insurance would not pay for them, her ear infections immediately returned along with the other symptoms.

"Before we went to the allergist, I had talked to several doctors. We had gone to the best doctors and to different children's hospitals. Their answers were operations for her ears and medication to help calm her down if necessary. After a while the doctors started to treat me like a neurotic mother, implying that I must be doing something wrong for my child to be doing this. Or else they said she was going through a phase and would grow out of it. Both those kinds of attitudes got very frustrating.

"This experience has taught me to trust myself. As a mother, you absolutely know your child, and if you feel that the physician you are talking to isn't correct, then you should question it, and go with your gut instinct because chances are you're probably right. As a parent, you know your child best. Since we've been working with Dr. Buttram, Brittany is doing much better, staying on the diet and avoiding foods to which she's sensitive. The main thing I would say is, 'Trust your instincts and keep looking until you find what works.'".

23. Attention Deficit Disorders

Attention deficit disorder is the term used to describe children with all kinds of learning problems and hyperactivity. As Dr. Michael Schachter notes, these conditions are frequently improved by cleaning up children's diets and removing fluoride: "Some of these children are sensitive to fluoride, which may cause headaches, hyperactivity, and problems with attention. Fluoride is often present in their drinking water and tooth paste! Some children are prescribed fluoride tablets or given fluoride treatments at their dentists' offices or at school. Some of these children are benefited by removing all sources of fluoride. Additionally, vitamin and mineral supplements, such as magnesium, may be quite helpful.

"Homeopathy can also be extremely useful for these children. I saw one little boy who suffered from recurrent ear infections and was hyperactive. When we gave him the proper homeopathic remedy, removed sugar from his diet, and gave him a little cod liver oil, the pediatricians and specialists who had been following him for his ear infections and asthma were amazed at how beautifully he did; he turned out not to require tubes in his ears, which they had recommended. Also, his attention deficit and concentration span improved."

"Tim:" A Personal Account of Attention Deficit Disorder

"I am the mother of Timothy, who is five years old. For five years I had been trying to find out what was wrong with Timothy. It's really been a personal battle. Many people looked at me cross-eyed and said that he is a normal little boy, he is just growing; or he is immature; or it is my fault because I don't discipline him properly; I am not stern enough, they said, and I should introduce physical punishment. Since Tim was my first child, I had nothing to compare his behavior to and since I was coming out of the corporate world, I didn't really know with whom I could share my doubts and insecurities. I felt very vulnerable exposing myself to other mothers and saying, 'I can't do this. What's wrong with my child?'

"By the time Tim was three, there were times when I just couldn't stand being a mother. All I did was say 'No, no, no' all the time. He started doing dangerous things to his younger brother, such as pushing him down the basement stairs in a walker. And I thought, 'This is not Timothy. He knows that that is not right.' There was a look in his eye, and I thought, 'What has possessed him to do this?' I just knew that something wasn't right and I was told that the reason why he was acting out in this way was because of his new brother, that this was typical, and not to worry, to discipline him as necessary.

"When he was four, his schoolteacher said, 'I'm having a difficult time with this child. He is extremely bright. He is conceptually aware of wrinkles and God and stars and things like that, but he can't color in the pictures and he doesn't know how to socialize with other children.' So I decided that it was time to go to a child behavior specialist who said that when he could sit still, Tim demonstrated a high IQ. However, they also said he was extremely immature and needed to be observed.

"By the time he turned five, his pre-kindergarten teacher said, 'He's a problem child and I suspect that he has an attention-deficit disorder, with hyperactive tendencies. I suggest that you get some medical care.' We brought him to the hospital and the behavior specialist said that Ritalin would be necessary at this point, along with some counseling.

"Based on our family history of chemical dependency, I felt that Ritalin was not a good option. So I started looking for other possibilities. That September, just two weeks after the diagnosis, we had a birthday party, and I served my boy ice cream, chocolate cake, and a glass of milk. And he went totally off the wall. In order to try to control him, I had the children play school because they all loved it. I asked him to recite his ABC's and he stopped at 'D.' Now he had known the whole alphabet for a year and he just panicked. He looked so scared, absolutely horrified. He said, 'Mommy, I don't know what to do. What comes after D, what comes after D?' I knew it was the food, and that from there I needed to find an answer.

"I happened to see a program with Doris Rapp on

the Phil Donohue Show, *and I picked up her book and read it. I gave my son the multiple-elimination diet that she suggested and the results were unbelievable! Even the pediatricians and the other doctors were surprised. In fact, the chief of the pediatric staff, who is also a personal friend, was extremely intrigued, but because of his position in the medical field and the way he was trained, he, at this point, wasn't able to offer me any medical support. But he did support my going to Dr. Buttram until he could learn more himself in this field. So here was the chief of the pediatric staff who was interested but unable to help me.*

"I've done a lot of reading and now realize that the majority of our M.D.'s have no nutritional background. Now that I have figured out that my son's problem is food allergies as well as allergies to environmental substances such as pollens, it really bothers me that medical doctors don't have this fundamental knowledge of nutrition. It would have been wonderful if, during those first five years, my doctor had been able to say, 'What do you feed your child? Have you noticed a pattern?'

"Now, in reviewing the first five years of Timothy's life, I notice a pattern. From the time he was one year old, he has always been at his worst during July and August. There was absolutely no dealing with him. I remember that because it was always before his check-up, and I was always going to the pediatrician and saying, 'I can't deal with this child. What is wrong with him?' And they would say that we would work out some behavior modification rules together. Now I realize he is severely allergic to

ragweed, to the grasses, and to dairy and corn. When he came in contact with these substances all at once, it just gave him a full-barrel effect. In the summertime we would eat fresh corn on the cob, and after, as a wonderful treat for the whole family, we'd jump in the car and go Dairy Queen, with all the ragweed blowing around. Now that was why I was dealing with a monster. As soon as the frost hit, he was much better.

"Now, after six months under Dr. Buttram's care, Timothy is a totally changed child. The school system is extremely interested and is keeping a file on him in the clinic, and they're suggesting to other parents that they go this route, because Tim now shows no symptoms of attention-deficit disorder. The kindergarten program he will be entering next year has already tested him and, in their opinion, he is a normal child and shows no evidence of an attention deficit. Plus there is no hyperactivity and has been none for at least four months."

24. Autism

Autism is a collection of symptoms usually characterized by a child's inability to use words for language, an absence of eye contact, and an inability to relate well to people—or even to objects. As Dr. Leander Ellis explains, "Little kids with autism don't play with toys; they are in a foggy cocoon of their own.

"An infant's brain is like a do-it-yourself kit that has to be built over a period of about 25 years," Dr. Ellis continues. "If you stop him at any point along the way, particularly in the first three years, you are going to have what we call an autistic child. If you stop him substantially beyond that, you get some attenuation but a child that is on a level that is much higher. If you stop the ones below the age of about three years, they tend to actually regress and lose some of the functions that they have already learned.

"I saw a four-and-a-half year old boy recently. His medical history showed that he had ear infections and multiple exposures to antibiotics, and that regression started around 20 months. Within two weeks after we put him on a milk-free and wheat-free diet, with no sugar and no obvious sources of mold or yeast, he began to talk and play with toys, to make eye contact, and to relate to other people. I put him on a mild anti-fungal agent and he regressed markedly. His mother cut down the dosage to about a quarter of how much I had given him, which was already a small dose, and in about ten days he brightened up. When he came back five weeks after the first evaluation, he walked in with a little spaghetti machine that he was pushing play dough into and cranking out play dough spaghetti, and he said, 'I'm making spaghetti.' He acted like a typical child, asking numerous questions of his parents about everything in the place. He had become a toy fanatic. They joined a toy-lending service, to meet his insatiable desire for toys.

"The child, who is now about six, is reading, drawing, and can sound out some words. He is still mildly hyperactive because he's reacting to the mold in the air, especially in the spring, but he is markedly improved. We also use nutritional support and his mother has him in an intensive tutoring program."

Dr. Sidney Baker offers additional insight into the nature of autism and the limits of our understanding of it. "All doctors are taught that if you get the right diagnosis, then you'll know the treatment for that person. My patient Jamie illustrates an essential problem with this belief. He was originally diagnosed as being autistic, and there was relatively little discussion questioning the accuracy of that diagnosis. He really exhibited the classic symptoms of autism. But to say that, because we know the diagnosis, we know the treatment for all the people in that illness group, is not a very useful approach. In Jamie, the pattern of biochemical abnormalities was not especially characteristic of autism. Jamie had a subset of problems that may go with that group, including disturbances of digestion (probably a disturbance of the germs that live in his digestive tract, which may be the mediators of the sugar response) and a bunch of other biochemical markers. My approach to treating him was simply to find everything that was out of balance and, keeping an open mind, to say, 'Let's measure as many things as are reasonable to do, step by step, and fix the imbalances where they occur.'

"I don't think that we entirely understand autism, even using this approach. I think that autism is the single most elusive diagnosis to make, at least in terms of finding the key to it. But when you approach children with what you could call this naive approach of fixing imbalances where you find them, it really works quite well. Part of the corrective action involves helping the child to stay away from things that he or she is bothered by—either foods to which he or she is allergic or sugars—and helping him or her get enough of the nutrients that seem to satisfy a particular biochemical need. Early intervention really helps a lot in the future of such children."

Dr. Michael Schachter describes some of the research currently being conducted in autism around the world. "There is some really good research, especially in France, that shows that magnesium and B_6 will help considerably—though not cure—autism, much more than some of the drugs that are commonly used, and with fewer side effects. Some ten or 12 double-blind, placebo-controlled studies have shown that magnesium and B_6 are helpful for autism in children. I'm working with one young man now who's autistic, and we seem to have run up against some interactions with some of the drugs that he was on (including Inderal and Haldol). But the controlled studies indicate that autism can be helped with magnesium and B_6. DMG, dimethylglycine, also seems to be helpful, not only with autism but also with reducing aggressive behavior."

"Jamie:" A Personal Account of Autism

"My son Jamie is now three-and-a-half years old. When he was about 15 months old, he began to lose a lot of the qualities seen in normal children. He stopped talking, he stopped interacting, and he stopped making eye contact. All of this began to point toward autism. Prior to that time, he had been very, very healthy and had developed well ahead of his milestones, except for a very long period of ear infections, which were treated by an equally long course of antibiotics. Over time, we became more and more concerned about him. At about 18 months, he was diagnosed with severe language delay, meaning that he was not doing anything that the average 18-month-old child does to communicate. Also, he had developed a number of rather bizarre behavioral traits, including spinning and staring at the walls and only playing by himself.

"We saw a child psychiatrist in Maryland where we live, who suggested that we did have a very serious problem but that he wasn't sure that it was autism. He wanted us to look into the possibility of allergies and yeast infection. So we found various people to address those issues and Jamie began to improve. As the improvement continued, he began to speak again, after about six months. But the improvement was somewhat limited. He still didn't interact with other children, even though a lot of the bizarre behavior had receded and he had perked up quite a bit.

"We were looking for further help with the allergies and the developmental problems because it still *seemed as though there was a missing piece. So in April 1992, we went to Princeton to see Dr. Baker. Dr. Baker has very thoroughly investigated Jamie's biochemistry and provided treatment and a lot of suggestions and support. Jamie experienced another big jump forward to the point that now his allergies are of relatively little concern, his development is almost on track (about six to eight months behind), and his behavior and his speech are vastly improved. In the fall, he will go to a normal nursery school, although the children will be six to eight months younger than he is. Aside from this, he will be back on track.*

"We realize that we are able to turn his symptoms on and off by simply modifying his diet, so we try to be careful with what we feed him. Sugar is the biggest offender. He can take it in very small amounts periodically. But if he gets too much of it, it is like shooting a rubber band across the room. He just flies around the house, becomes totally unreasonable, somewhat destructive, and very aggressive. He also becomes overly emotional. He realizes that we are going to try to discipline him for acting out, even though he is aware that his behavior is not really within his control. So I think he feels unjustly persecuted when he is punished."

25. Behavioral Disorders

Dr. Harold Buttram describes how behavioral disorders in children, such as hyperactivity, are caused by chemicals, and the history of successfully identifying and treating the problem:

"If you spend an hour in a room with a full-blown hyperactive child, you will never forget it. These kids are literally off the wall. They are constantly moving, as they are incapable of spending concentrated attention on any given task, even playing. They're irritable and very often aggressive and hostile. Doris Rapp has shown pictures of some of these children biting their mothers, trying to destroy toys, and this sort of thing. These are extremely disturbed children.

"Parents often use the term Jekyll-and-Hyde to describe their children. When they're doing well they may be sweet and lovable little children. Then, if they eat something to which they're allergic, very often a junk food, you get the Jekyll-and-Hyde transformation. They become ugly and belligerent.

"What actually happens here is the cerebral cortex, the higher center of the brain, literally shuts down and control gets thrown back to the more primitive centers. There is a center at the base of the brain, for instance, that has been shown to be a center for anger. What stimulates this center? Chemicals."

Dr. Buttram points out the link between an increase in environmental toxins over the years and a corresponding increase in behavioral disorders in children. "It is important to point out that there has been a drastic increase in behavioral disorders in children since World War II. Dr. William Crook, a retired pediatrician from Jackson, Tennessee, commented in a talk that when he went into practice as a pediatrician in the early 1950s he never saw a hyperactive child. I think people of my generation—I went to school in the 30s—in thinking back don't remember seeing a child with the hyperactive syndrome.

"It is really an ominous situation. I talked with a psychologist consultant for our school district not long ago and mentioned this subject. She stated that she has noticed among children increasing evidence of autistic tendencies. This is something that she has never really seen before. Thinking it might possibly be a local problem, she called other school districts and found they were observing the same thing.

"What has happened in the past 50 years that has brought about this increase in behavior disorders? According to published reports, before World War II, less than one billion pounds a year of organic chemicals were produced in the United States. By 1963, that number had increased to 163 billion pounds per year. Today it is somewhere around 250 billion pounds per year.

"According to an official publication, approximately 70,000 chemical compounds are now in commercial use. Of these, only about ten percent have had any testing at all for neurotoxicity. Among this ten percent, only a handful have had thorough testing.

"An interesting study was performed on residents of North Carolina, North Dakota, and New Jersey. The investigation

194

assayed the chemicals in indoor air, drinking water, and exhaled breath of 400 subjects. Ten volatile chemicals were found to be present in the exhaled breaths of most patients. These chemicals are therefore extremely prevalent.

"Organic volatile chemicals are lipid or fat soluble. Therefore, they have an affinity for the fatty or lipid tissues of the body. The brain is a primary target because it consists largely of lipid or fatty tissues. It is also a target because of its rich blood supply.

"The primary symptoms of volatile organic compounds are therefore cerebral. They include headaches, dizziness, difficulty with concentration, memory lapses, feelings of fogginess or spaciness, drowsiness, and fatigue.

"It's important to point out that in your standard text of neurotoxicology one of the earliest signs of chemical toxicity is that of behavioral changes. Therefore, I think there are very good reasons for tying in environmental chemicals with the epidemic we're having of behavioral problems such as attention deficit disorder and hyperactivity. The massive increase of environmental chemicals to which these children are exposed is connected to their symptoms.

"A combination of subtle brain damage from environmental chemicals, nutritional deficiencies, a crippling of the detoxification systems of the body, food allergies, and an overgrowth of candida in the system will produce a very sick child. The manifestation of this will be a crippled immune system. This means the child will have more allergies. He or she will be sick a lot of the time and on antibiotics. The brain function cannot possibly be normal; it would be a miracle if it were. The hyperactivity, attention deficit, and behavioral problems, in my opinion, are all actually a continued spectrum of the same thing."

Dr. Buttram identifies several specific groups of environmental chemicals. "Environmental chemicals fall into two general categories. One consists of toxic heavy metals, of which lead, of course, is the best known. This category would also include mercury, cadmium, aluminum, and others. Our concern here is more with the other category, the volatile organic compounds, which are made up of carbon molecules. The commercial uses of volatile compounds break down into three major classes: formaldehyde, organic solvents, and pesticides.

"Formaldehyde is present in many, many commercial products. It is present in new homes in the building materials, paneling, floors, and ceilings made of plywood or particle board. It's also present in the carpets, fixtures, and furnishings. The bad thing about formaldehyde in a building is that it is very slow to dissipate. Its half-life may be six, seven, or even ten years. It takes this long before it is dissipated to the point at which the building is safe to live in. Formaldehyde is also used in fabrics and is found in many of the clothes we wear.

"Organic solvents are present in hundreds, if not thousands, of products. They are commonly used in commercial items that we use all the time at home. They're found in perfumes made from synthetic musks, for instance, and in caulking, paint, varnishes, and cleaning solutions, which are often very toxic.

"Pesticides, our last category, may be the most dangerous of all. They are used, of course, to exterminate in homes or out of doors. If you live in a farm or orchard area you may be subject to pesticide drifts. There are also often significant residues in foods, especially in foods imported from countries where there is no regulation in the use of pesticides."

The treatment of the wide range of illnesses arising from

environmental chemicals, according to Dr. Buttram, must include education, enhanced nutrition, and nutritional supplements. "The pioneers in this field used to be called clinical ecologists, but they've now changed their name to the American Academy of Environmental Medicine. These are the people who have really broken ground in this area. They're leagues and leagues ahead of the more conventional medical doctors, and they've set the standard for several of the approaches to treatment we recommend.

"First, we educate parents on how to avoid chemicals. For virtually all of them this is a first, because nobody has ever talked to them about these things before. Identifying and eliminating poisons in the home is not usually that difficult. We take a history of the home environment in regard to the building of the home and other possible sources of chemical exposure to the child. We teach parents how to reduce exposure to the more toxic chemicals, such as formaldehyde and volatile sprays.

"The problems that arise often occur due to exposure in school. If you have a cooperative school administration, the problems can usually be solved. But from what I have seen, school staff and administration don't usually recognize the potential hazards to children of chemical exposure and their ignorance of the risks sometimes presents additional obstacles.

"Second, we do nutritional counseling in which we emphasize just plain simple food without chemicals. I detest the term 'health foods' because it's so misleading. I think 'plain foods' is a better term. I ask parents, who are now in their 30s and 40s, to think back about how their grandparents ate two generations ago. In many instances their wasn't ideal, but it was vastly superior to the way people eat today. They ate mostly plain, unadulterated food.

"So the prime emphasis in diet is the avoidance of chemicals. I attended a meeting in Dallas one time where William Rea was the speaker. He is certainly one of the most highly respected men today in the field of environmental medicine. Dr. Rea said that it's secondary whether a person is a vegetarian or a meat eater. What is far more important today is the avoidance of chemicals—both chemical additives and residual chemicals.

"In our area there are new markets called Fresh Fields that specialize in organic foods. If you're fortunate enough to live near markets such as these you can shop there, especially for organic fresh fruits and vegetables. Doctor's Data has some very good studies showing that organically grown food compared to market food has significantly higher levels of nutrient minerals and lower levels of toxic metals. Eating organic food, then, may be the most important thing of all. Beyond that, you need to focus on balanced nutrition.

"For children I think it is imperative to get organic fruits and fruit juices even if you can't do anything more than this. From the figures I've seen, fruit and fruit juice tend to be more highly contaminated with pesticide residues than other classes of foods. Children eat more fruit and drink by far more fruit juice than adults. From this source alone, they could very easily ingest toxic levels of pesticide residues.

"There was a book published recently called *Pesticides in the Diets of Infants and Children*, sponsored by the highly prestigious National Research Council, which is one of the highest government scientific advisory boards. This book, although scientifically written, really raised Cain about our present screening processes for pesticides and didn't mince words about it either. It claimed that the uncontrolled exposure of our children to these pesticide residues is highly prevalent.

"Third, for practically all children, we recommend a high-quality hypoallergenic multiple vitamin. We use one by Klaire Labs, which makes vitamins separate from minerals. We don't recommend giving large doses. We offer other nutritional supplements in special situations. When candida is present from antibiotic overuse, lactobacillus acidophilus and bifidus are given. When lead and other toxic heavy metals are found, we add a very simple detoxification component to the program, which includes vitamin C and garlic. Garlic is added because it is high in the sulfhydryl amino acids.

"We recommend using a high-quality flaxseed oil. This provides the essential fatty acids for the development of the brain, nervous system, and cell membranes. We emphasize nutrient minerals such as calcium and zinc since we know that these minerals can replace the toxic metals in the body. We particularly recommend beans and lentils, which are also high in sulfhydryl amino acids, because of their detoxification potential. The sulfur in these amino acids actually binds with the lead or other toxic heavy metals and helps to carry them out of the body.

"Food allergy testing is another important component," Dr. Buttram concludes. "Most of these children are allergic to certain foods and some of their major symptom complexes can be related to their food allergies. We can approach this either through elimination diets or else through skin testing, which we commonly do. We find neutralizing doses and treat with sublingual drops. This can work very well. When it does work you have some very grateful parents."

"Maria:" A Personal Account of a Behavioral Disorder

"My daughter, Maria, has been helped in a dramatic way by alternative medical approaches. A couple of months ago, Maria became wildly uncontrollable. She's only nine years old, but she was going out at five and six o'clock in the morning to shop with homeless people. She would go into violent rages and would sleep only about four or five hours a night. Finally, I couldn't keep her home anymore and so I put her into a psychiatric hospital where they determined that she was suffering from manic depression. They started her on lithium but she wasn't herself; she wasn't conversational the way she usually is, and she was still depressed. She had elevated liver enzymes which, at the hospital, they failed to follow up on. She also had elevated levels of thyroid hormone, which they also failed to follow up on. After three weeks in the hospital, she had calmed down somewhat, and I was able to take her home. She still wasn't well.

"I had been consulting with Dr. Slagle while Maria was in the hospital because I have the utmost respect for her and knew that if anyone could figure out what was wrong with my daughter, she could. As soon as Maria came out of the hospital, she had several blood tests done, which showed she had antibodies against her thyroid and that her thyroid levels were fluctuating up and down. Also, she had probably had some sort of liver virus that had precipitated this auto-immune reaction in her thyroid. Dr. Slagle prescribed amino acids, B vitamins, and several other vitamins, as well as a

homeopathic cortisone and baby aspirin to help shrink the swelling of her thyroid.

"On the second day of her taking the aspirin and the homeopathic cortisone, her behavior became completely normal. It was a miracle. For close to a month and a half, my daughter had been completely out of control, unable to have a conversation, alternating between being hysterical and being completely quiet. I had been so terrified. It was as if I had lost her. And on the second day of the medication, she began to be able to hold conversations; she was completely normal—like herself again. I know that had I not gone to Dr. Slagle, she would have continued on lithium and been somewhat controllable, but not herself.

"Dr. Slagle also found that she was highly allergic. My daughter had very allergic reactions to various foods that she was eating on a regular basis. It was clear that her problem had been her immune system and not a psychiatric disorder, which never would have been taken care of had she just stuck with traditional medical doctors, even though she was being seen by some of the best in the country. So thanks to Dr. Slagle and the alternative medical field in general, I have my daughter back."

26. Chronic Depression

Just as Dr. Leander Ellis insisted that more children today suffer from behavioral disorders than in the past, Dr. Lendon Smith asserts that more children today suffer from chronic depression. And like Dr. Ellis, Dr. Smith also cites the toxic overload created by environmental chemicals as the cause. Dr. Smith is particularly adamant about the importance of magnesium, and the magnesium deficiencies that have occurred in many children as a result of environmental poisoning.

"Today there are more children who are chronically depressed than there were in the past," begins Dr. Smith. "Our chemistry seems to indicate that chemical deficiencies are involved, e.g., magnesium deficiencies. Mr. Kitkoski, the chemist from Spokane, Washington, whose research I've shared, has spent a lot of time studying the function of electrolytes in the human body. He figured out that we all need the right amount of electrolytes to act as a buffering capacity for the blood. The electrolytes—sodium, potassium, bicarbonate, chloride, a little bit of sulfur, a little bit of magnesium, and some calcium—are all the things that become electrically active when they are dissolved.

Electrolytes have to do with controlling the pH, the acid/base balance, which controls what the minerals are doing, which brings us back to magnesium levels.

"I think that all the artificial chemicals that are in our environment and food are exerting a toxic overload on children. It's not just lead, but all the things that we are inhaling and eating, that are in our water, and all the things that are in our food that shouldn't be there, as well as the things that are removed from our food that we need. All these things are having an effect on our children.

"For example, I've visited classes of 25 or 30 children sitting there, restless, shuffling their feet, and I ask, 'How many of you have headaches once or twice a week?' and every hand goes up. I look around and see this sea of pale faces with circles under their eyes, as if they had all just been hit in the stomach. I ask them what they had for breakfast, and while they all said that they had eaten breakfast, it turns out to have been a donut or some other cake or pastry because their parents had no time to fix them a decent meal. Or, if the parents did fix them a decent meal, they wouldn't eat it anyway because they chose to get some candy on the way to school instead.

"I used to speak at the Reading Teachers Association meeting in California every year. Three thousand reading teachers would get together and have a meeting to decide what textbooks and what reading method they would use. They always had their meeting in the first week in November because they all knew they couldn't teach any of the kids until all the Halloween candy had been eaten. The kids were just . . . gone! So teachers certainly know about children's poor eating habits.

"Stephen Schoenthaler, a sociology professor at the University of California, did an experiment from 1979 to 1984 with almost a million New York City school kids. The kids were given breakfast and lunch, without sugar, color, or flavor additives. Over a period of five years, the achievement scores of the children went up significantly—without a change in the teaching methods. Only the diet had been changed. The kids who were getting the best grades at the end of those five years were the kids who were eating the school foods, so the researchers knew they could have a positive impact with diet. Obviously diet isn't the whole answer to educational problems, but it's a start," Dr. Smith concludes.

27. Food Allergies

When people think of child allergies they think of hay fever, asthma, eczema, and hives. But there are many other areas of the body that can be affected by allergies. As Dr. Doris Rapp informs us, "Allergies can cause headaches or stomachaches; they can affect the bladder, causing your child to wet the bed or to have to run to get to the toilet in time. Allergies can cause leg aches, muscle aches, joint aches, sleep problems, behavior problems, and learning problems. Some children will become tense, nervous, and irritable. Others will become withdrawn and unreachable, hiding in corners and pulling away when you go to touch them. Still others will become very hyperactive and aggressive. Often they will bite, hit, scream, and do all kinds of nasty things.

"Most allergists—including myself for my first 18 years in practice—would not recognize this host of physical and emotional symptoms as having been caused by allergies. But I now recognize that dust, molds, pollens, foods, and chemicals can affect almost any area of the body and can cause all of the problems mentioned above in some individuals.

"Now it would be going too far to suspect that every time a child has a headache it is an allergic reaction, or that every time an adult has a bellyache it is due to food sensitivity. But currently, with conventional medical practitioners, this diagnosis is never even considered and is therefore missed too many times. People will have headaches for years and never once consider whether there might some underlying reason for the headache.

"Environmental medicine wants patients to start to take more control of their health. We want you to pay attention to how you feel. If you don't feel well, or you suddenly can't think correctly; if you're confused, or unusually irritable, or emotionally volatile; if you cry or become upset or angry for no reason; you have to start to ask, 'Why am I having this reaction now? What did I eat, touch, or smell?' Our whole society is geared to go to the medicine cabinet for a painkiller or an antihistamine when we should be geared to get a pencil and paper to record what could be causing this problem at this time.

"After we have educated the parents, they often come in to see us knowing exactly what is causing their child's problems. They can tell if it's something inside or outside the house, if it's a food or a chemical. They can pinpoint the cause.

"Basically, why would a child have allergies or environmental illness? One of the main reasons is that their immune system is not up to par. If the immune system is inadequate, we can develop allergies and environmental illness. One way to strengthen the immune system so that your child is less prone to environmental illness or allergy is by using various nutrients. A helpful resource is the book, *Super Immunity in Kids*, which says, basically: If you take the correct nutrients in the correct amounts, you can strengthen the immune system so that you are less apt to become ill from natural things such as pollen, dust, and mold exposures.

You will also be less apt to become ill from exposure to infections.

"Now how can a parent tell if their child's learning problems are related to environmental factors? Think back. Does your child say, 'When I go to school in the morning I feel great!'? Or does the child say, 'I feel great when I leave the house and by the time I get to school I don't feel right.'? Or does he say, 'I feel nervous'? Or tired, or irritable, or, 'I have a headache.'? If that happens, you have to think, it might be the fumes on the school bus, or what he ate for breakfast, or what he uses to brush his teeth, or the soap that he uses. You've got to think of everything that he came in contact with before he got on the bus, and then what happened when he was on the bus.

"One way for parents to figure out what's causing the problem is to drive the child to school. If you find he can eat, bathe, wash, and do everything else in the usual manner in the morning and you drive him to school and he's fine, then it's probably the bus that is causing problems. And you can check back and forth a couple of times and try to confirm or negate your suspicions. Now, children who are sensitive to things in the school will frequently notice that their headache starts within an hour. And the headaches frequently become more intense during the day. By Friday afternoon, the headache will be much worse than it was on Monday morning or on Sunday night. At first the headaches may disappear one to four hours after your child leaves school, but later on, if there are too many exposures during the week, you may notice that they don't get better at night and that it might take the whole weekend for the headache to go away.

"Another clue that certain exposures are making your child feel worse is when your child can smell everything before anybody else. She smells natural gas, or smells that perfume across the room, or she can smell food cooking before anybody else. She can smell disinfectants. If these odors bother your child and she can perceive them faster than anybody else, it means that she is probably becoming sensitized to the abundance of chemicals that we have now managed to put in our food, air, water, clothing, homes, schools, and workplaces.

"What else do you notice if a child is sensitive to something in school? The child may get an A one day, and an F the next day in the same subject. It isn't that your child lost brain cells within 24 hours, but it does indicate to me that you should investigate that school to try to find out what could be causing the problem. Is the school dusty or moldy? Are the ventilation ducts open and clean? Was the basement of the school ever flooded? Does it smell worse on damp days? There is nothing worse in present-day schools than some of the synthetic carpets. They are made of chemicals that cause problems. In addition, they use adhesives that are full of other chemicals that cause even more problems. Many of these chemicals are neurotoxic, which means they damage the nervous system, or carcinogenic, which means they can cause cancer.

"Here is a list of symptoms you may recognize from your child's behavior: The ability to hear, talk, or speak clearly is impaired. Your child suddenly speaks too fast—is hyperactive—or doesn't make sense when he talks. An environmental sensitivity can alter children's ability to write, read, or see clearly. Some children develop blurred vision or double vision by the end of the day because of chemical exposures at school. Some develop red earlobes or cheeks, wriggly legs or dark circles under their eyes. All of these signs and symptoms can be caused by an environmental illness.

"If you suspect that your child may have been exposed to neurotoxic substances—those that actually damage the nervous system—ask your doctor to send you to specialists who can tell you whether the nerve conduction time in your child's body is normal or not. They can do a variety of blood tests to find out if the chemicals that are in the carpets and the adhesives are in the blood.

"The doctor may even make an allergy extract of the air in a room that smells of chemicals. Sometimes the child is exposed to just one drop of the allergy extract of the air of a room—a particular room in the home or school—we can actually reproduce a headache, a stomachache, or problems thinking. The doctor makes the allergy extract the same way one would bubble air through a fish tank: Using a pump to bubble the room air through a salt solution in a tiny test tube. The air bubbles for about eight hours and at the end of this period a solution remains that contains some of the chemicals that were in the air. Then an allergy extract is prepared from this solution which can be injected in the skin, or placed under the tongue. If it causes numbness in the arms, tingling in the fingers, a headache, stomachache, problems with remembering, or a change in activity or behavior within ten minutes, we have probably collected the problem chemical from the air within the solution.

"Using the new and more precise method of allergy testing called provocation/neutralization, the doctor can then make dilutions of that chemical solution and probably eliminate those same symptoms with one drop of the right dilution of that solution. In other words, if the child develops a headache in a certain room, you can put a drop of the air allergy extract under the tongue and provoke the headache in three to eight minutes. Then you can give the child a five-fold weaker dilution of that same solution and often you can eliminate or neutralize the headache in less than ten minutes.

"After you have done a skin test with the allergy extracts, and shown that there is a cause-and-effect relationship between the child's behavior or physical symptoms and a chemical in the school, the next thing is to determine what the school can do to eliminate the problem. One of the things they can do is not put carpets in schools. If they do have carpets and they're causing problems, they can take the carpets up and put in hard vinyl tile. In such cases, it is important to insist that they use adhesives that are safe when installing the tile.

"Another big problem in schools is poor ventilation, especially in the winter. Due to the energy crunch we had in the '70s, many schools closed down their ventilation systems to save money and to cut down on the cost of heating. Dust, molds, and chemicals have accumulated at very high levels in these schools. The windows don't always open, and the result is that there has been a gradual build-up, so that more and more children and teachers seem to be adversely affected when they go to school.

"One of the things that you can insist on is that school officials check the ventilation system. There are fast and easy ways to measure the amount of carbon dioxide in a classroom, which can tell you whether the ventilation is good or not. The level should be 800 ppm or less. Relatively simple tests can also be done to measure for certain chemicals, such as chlorine and formaldehyde. Sometimes, because of poor cleaning of the ventilation systems in schools, the problem is dust and molds, not chemicals. Other times, they put chemicals in the ductwork while cleaning, which really causes trouble because the chemicals then circulate throughout the school, causing illness. Sometimes the intake for the ventilation system is too close to the area where all the school buses line up. The bus drivers let the engines idle for long periods, resulting in all the gasoline fumes and hydrocarbons entering the ductwork intake and circulating throughout the school.

"In one case I encountered, a school had a printing press, and the exhaust pipe from the printing press was at exactly the same level as the ventilation intake on the roof, with the result that all the chemicals from the printing press were going right back in and circulating throughout the school. Some printing press chemicals are toxic to the nervous system and cancer-causing.

"A patient I saw last week has three sons who came home smelling of mop oil, which is used to clean the school. The mother said that the children's clothes smelled so badly that she had to use very hot water to eliminate the smell. One of the boys developed a headache and a burning sensation in his throat. So I asked her to bring some of the mop oil and I just put it underneath his nose and let him take one whiff of the odor. Within seconds, he was complaining of a headache around his forehead on both sides of his temples and he said it was throbbing and that his throat was burning. I gave him oxygen for about ten minutes and the headache, throbbing, and burning in his throat gradually subsided. We videotaped this reaction.

"There was another child who had trouble only on the two afternoons a week when he went to school. He would be weak and tired, hardly able to stand; he couldn't hold a pencil, clung to his mother, but only on those two days. I sent the mother to the school and asked her to try to figure out what's different in the schoolroom that might be causing your son problems. It turned out that they used a very common disinfectant aerosol in the room, six times a day on the tabletops, to reduce infections. Then they used the same solution on the cot that he napped on. All she had to do was ask the school to stop using that disinfectant and install an air purifier, and the child improved remarkably.

"Then the mother noticed that he had similar problems when he went into the gym, and it turned out that they were using a certain kind of floor wax in the gym. We suggested that they use something that had fewer petrochemicals in it and the result was that he can now be in the gym for 20 minutes. That child had tics and twitches, which is another thing that you see in some children with these allergies. The symptoms disappeared after environmental allergy care.

"I have seen children from all over the country who have problems at school. Some of these children who come to see me don't come in complaining of allergies. But the affected teachers and the children almost uniformly have a history of hay fever, asthma, or eczema. And they have relatives that have these same conditions. Their immune systems are not up to par, or they wouldn't have allergies to start with. But they are the canaries— the first ones to become ill when a school is chemically contaminated, or is too dusty or too moldy. Many children who have these allergies also find that their problems grow worse after their school has been remodeled, repainted, newly carpeted, or refurnished with furniture made of materials that release formaldehyde or other chemicals into the air.

"Children who wheezed a little before, now wheeze a lot. Youngsters who were stuffy once in a while are now congested all the time. Not only do they get nose problems, but they start having infections in the sinuses and their ears. Many of them feel tired and weak when the schools are chemically contaminated. One parent said that their child was too tired to turn the pages of his book. Another said that her child was crying because he couldn't play football anymore because he was just too weak. These are some of the things that are happening in some schools throughout the country, mainly because of dust, molds, and chemicals.

"Schools also serve food, and much of the food is contaminated with pesticides. Ideally, your child should eat only organically grown food because it is less contaminated with pesticides, food coloring, or other chemical additives that may be causing your child's adverse reactions. However, in some places, it remains difficult—and expensive—to buy foods uncontaminated by chemicals. Organic foods may be readily available in New York City, but they certainly aren't in many other cities. I encourage people to grow their own vegetables so that they will have their own source in the winter and one which they know does not contain any chemicals.

"There is one very important and simple thing you can do to tell which area in a school or in your home, or which food, might be causing your children a problem. Ask your children how they feel before they eat a meal, or before they enter a particular room. Also ask them to write their name and to draw. You should do the same thing. And then, if you have asthma, blow into something called a Peak Pocket Flow Meter, which is a plastic tube with a gauge on it. If you blow 400 before you eat and half an hour later you blow 200, one or more of the foods that you ate is causing asthma or spasm of your lungs. Check out each food separately five days later and find the culprit.

"Another thing to do is to take your child's pulse before eating. If the pulse is 80 and suddenly after eating it is 120, a food has set off a silent alarm in the child's body, which has caused her pulse to increase. So check the writing, the drawing, the pulse rate, the breathing, and how your child feels and looks before a meal and then a half hour or so later. If any of these variables indicates a change for the worse after a meal, one of the foods your child ate may be the cause of the problem. If the change occurs after being in a particular room or area, something in there may be at cause.

"Wait for five days before the attempt to find the problem food. It is critical that you wait for five days to get all that particular food out of the body. So for five days, if you have noticed your child had a reaction after eating corn, don't feed your child corn (and tell her not to eat any at school either). Then at eight a.m. on a Saturday, give her the first of the foods she may have been reacting to, and at ten a.m. give her the second possibility one, at noon the next one, and at one p.m. the next. In this way, you check each food all by itself. Again, check the breathing, the pulse, the writing and drawing, and how your child feels and looks before and a half hour or so after each food.

"You can apply the same principles of food isolation to every room in your house and at school or every room at work. Check your breathing (or your child's breathing) before you enter a room, do all the things that I suggested above, and then do them again several hours later. If you find that a particular room is a problem, then you have got to ask, 'Why? What do I smell in this room, what am I touching in this room, what is in this room that could be bothering me? Is it the heating system, the covering on the furniture, the carpet, the floor wax, the furniture polish? Are there items that have been dry-cleaned in this room? Is there an odor?' You'll be surprised at how much you can figure out on your own.

"Also check out the car. Notice how you and your children feel before you get in the car, then check again half an hour later. Compare indoors with outdoors and you'll be able to tell whether it's the outdoor pollution, the lawn spray next door, the mold, pollen, or pollution in the air that is causing problems outside versus inside. You can easily figure out many, many answers by checking your child's pulse, his breathing, and how he writes, draws, feels and looks. Check these same parameters on yourself as well. If you have high blood pressure, you can even use a blood pressure cuff and check your pressure before and after each of these exposures and you'll turn up answers. By keeping detailed records, you can often figure out the reasons why your children are ill, and many times you can then get rid of the cause and make them feel much better.

"Don't forget to check lavatories. Many children go into the lavatories at school feeling fine, and when they come out they can't think at all because of the chemicals in the disinfectants and deodorants that are used in the lavatories. Don't forget the garage, which has many chemicals in it. Don't forget the attic, which is dusty, and don't forget the basement, which is dusty and moldy.

"Keep in mind: The indoor and outdoor factor that causes more problems than any other is molds. If you live in a moldy house and you are always wheezing, on cortisone, always sick and in and out of the hospital, it could be the moldy house that you are living in that is causing the problem. Sometimes if you live in too much mold, it doesn't matter what kind of treatment you're on. You have to move or get away from the thing that is causing the problems.

"In the workplace, don't forget all the areas that have chemicals which could be affecting your brain. Remember: Excessive chemical exposures can and will damage the body. If they can't be excreted, they can be stored in the fat, and sometimes these fatty tissues get an overload and develop cancer. When you breathe something, these chemicals can go straight through your nose, right up into your brain. There is no barrier there to protect your brain. And the brain is, to a large degree, fat.

"There are some new ways of doing brain imaging that can actually show changes in the brains of some of the people that are exposed to neurotoxic substances. For example, if a child sniffs glue or hair spray or aerosols, you can actually show a characteristic pattern of change in the brain imaging-pattern on the particular individual, which will look different from somebody who has epilepsy or someone who has schizophrenia or depression. They actually produce different brain pictures. I'm sure in a few years, many people who say they are always depressed, or tired, or nervous will be able to have a brain-image pattern taken that will show that specific areas of the brain have been affected by certain exposures or foods.

"Ask your children to write down or tell you their five favorite foods and beverages. The five foods and beverages that they write are probably the foods that are most likely to cause them difficulty. If they wrote down chocolate, cocoa, and cola—which are all different forms of chocolate—it means that chocolate could be the cause of their problems. If they wrote down bread, cake, cookies, pasta, and macaroni, chances are the problem is wheat. If they wrote down ice cream, yogurt, milk, cheese, and pizza, they are probably sensitive to dairy products. In fact, the food that causes more chronic and acute illness in all of society, to my mind, is, unquestionably, milk and dairy products," Dr. Rapp concludes.

"Alison:" A Personal Account of Food Allergies

"As Alison's mother, I can honestly say that Alison was born crying. She cried for the first two years of her life. I took her to a clinic at the time and found out she was allergic to corn, wheat, and bananas, which caused her to cry every day, all day long. I

took her off those foods, and she became a normal, happy two-year-old. She did well for quite a while until she got a problem with a vitamin deficiency, which caused her to be uncontrollable. I couldn't do anything with her. If I wanted her to get dressed she would scream, rant, and rave. It would take me three hours just to get her dressed. After reading an article on vitamins, I put her on vitamin supplements. That's when we realized that she hadn't smiled in six months. Then she was fine again, until two years ago, when she started to scream at me all the time, day in and day out, no matter what I wanted her to do, over absolutely nothing. She would scream at me that her shoes were wrong, her hair was wrong. It would take me all day long just to get her into the shower. At this point she was ten years old. She should have been bathing on her own. I would go pick her up at school and when she was 70 feet away from me, she would scream, 'Mom, you are early!' And she would go on and on about why I was early. The next day she'd look at me and she'd scream, 'Mom, you are late!' And she would scream the whole way home, until she went up to her room and I would go off somewhere else to get away from her. She got worse and worse all summer, and in the fall, almost two years ago, I took her to Dr. Buttram.

"Dr. Buttram diagnosed my daughter as having food allergies: to corn, potatoes, chicken, egg yolks, rice, and chocolate. They put her on these sublingual drops and now I have my normal, happy daughter back again. It was a dramatic change. She had become extremely difficult to live with. She would

just scream at me about the most ridiculous things. Nothing was ever right. If she got out of bed—Why didn't I wake her up?—Why didn't I let her sleep?— And she would shriek at the top of her lungs. Some days were worse than others. Now I know that on the days she had a combination of foods or a lot of the foods she was allergic to that she was at her worst. The way that I figured out it was food again was because every once in awhile we would have a great day or two and every once in awhile her diet just happened to not include these things. Then she would be fine. But the next day she'd be right back again with the behavior—totally out of control for long periods of time.

"When my mother found out about Alison's behavior, she told me that I myself had been an absolutely horrendous child. Now that Alison had been diagnosed, she understood that I had had food allergies too. Now I understand that children's behavior problems are not always due to what the parent is doing with the child, as far as discipline is concerned. I've had a lot of children; I've been a foster parent for years. When Alison first started this behavior I tried everything in the book and nothing worked. And the thing that told me that something was controlling her, instead of her doing this, was the fact that we would have good days. And it didn't matter what we were doing on a bad day. If I would sit and play with her all day long, and it was a bad day, we would have a bad day. And discipline meant absolutely nothing, because something was controlling Alison. It was a chemical imbalance in her brain that was controlling her because she had

absolutely no control over what she did. It was like the food was controlling her. I related it to the behavior of a manic-depressive or a paranoid schizophrenic who has no control over what they are doing.

"Now, when I go to the shopping mall, I see kids who I know have food allergies by the way they are crying. My husband used to say I was crazy, but when Alison was two years old and she would cry, I could tell if it was a food-allergy cry or a two-year-old cry by the sound of her voice. It was a different kind of crying. I have friends who complain about their kids constantly and one child in particular I know has food allergies. And the mother will not take him in to be tested. She'd rather complain about it. The biggest obstacle I see to helping children with behavior problems caused by allergies is making parents understand that there is an alternative. You don't have to live like this. You have to ask yourself, 'Do I really want my child to live like this?'

"I feel bad that Alison was so miserable for so long. There are so many kids out there that are this miserable. There are kids in learning disability classes and the parents just don't look any further than their nose. Some parents do make an effort and take their kids to standard allergists who test them, but those doctors may not be able to locate the problem. A friend of mine took her child to a regular allergist who tested him for all the standard things and said he was fine. But he never tested him for half the things to which Alison is allergic and the doctor never questioned the mother about the child's diet."

28. Hyperactivity

Dr. Lendon Smith summarizes some of the history of treating hyperactivity in children, and then describes his own clinical experience: "The man who discovered the paradoxical effects of stimulant drugs on hyperactive children was Charles Bradley from Portland, Oregon. In 1937 and 1938, he found that most children with 'hyperactive syndrome' came from difficult pregnancies, especially those which ended in troublesome deliveries. The hyperactive children were the second of twins or born with the cord around their neck. They were premature, or born with a collapsed lung or too much bilirubin. A number of things might have interfered with the oxygen supply to the brain. The problems had not been enough to hurt the child's intellect but just enough to hurt the part of the brain that has to do with self-control. This was Bradley's original concept.

"Then, in 1938, a mistake was made. Charles Bradley was in charge of a home for problem children when he asked a nurse to give an overly active girl some bromide. The nurse accidentally used the next bottle, Benzedrine, and the girl promptly went to sleep. The doctor commented to the nurse that the bromide sure worked well and the nurse responded by saying, 'What did you say?' The doctor asked, 'What did you give her?' It turned out that this was the first time anybody had ever used a stimulant drug on somebody who already seemed to be overstimulated. That started the seemingly paradoxical treatment approach of giving stimulants to hyperactive children.

"Researchers have since found that the part of the brain primarily affected in hyperactive children is the limbic system. Hyperactive children don't seem to have enough norepinephrine, a brain neurotransmitter, in their limbic system in the little cells that have to do with inhibitory control. That's why Ritalin, Dexedrine, Benzedrine, caffeine to a certain extent, and some other stimulant drugs have a calming effect on these children. They prevent the reuptake of norepinephrine at the synaptic cleft. This is something all neurologists understand.

"I was working with a lot of hyperactive children in my practice in Oregon," Dr. Smith continues. "One of the children I was treating was affected by this syndrome. We found that speed, methamphetamine, was helpful to her. Teachers would send children they suspected of having the syndrome to me.

"I began to notice that these children had certain traits in common. They had short attention spans and they were unable to disregard unimportant stimuli. Everything came into their nervous system from their eyes, their ears, their skin, and their muscles with equal intensity. They were unable to selectively respond to certain stimuli and to ignore others. They couldn't just pay attention to the teacher, the board, or what was in their workbook.

"We found that many of these children would calm down after being placed on five or ten mg of Ritalin or Dexedrine. If they responded we diagnosed them as having the hyperactive syndrome. If that didn't work then we believed something else to be wrong.

"We had trouble ruling out psychological disorders or problems at home. You can imagine these children disrupting not only the classroom but the home environment as well, resulting in their parents either beating them or finding some other rigid disciplinary measure in their attempts to get these children to settle down and pay attention. Over a period of ten years I saw seven or eight thousand of these children and I noticed a pattern that interested me. I found a ratio of 5:1, boys:girls. This rules out Dr. Bradley's theory that hyperactivity was a result of a hurt to the nervous system. If he was right the ratio would have been 50/50.

"I also found these children to be fair most of the time. They were blue-eyed blondes and green-eyed redheads. We did see some Afro-Americans but in general they were fair-headed and light-skinned. I concluded that some genetic factors were involved here. I also discovered that these hyperactive children generally were very ticklish, goosey, sensitive. When I shined a light in their ears to check their eardrums, the light would bother them as if they could hear a light and see sounds. It was incredible how sensitive they were. The stethoscope was always cold on their chest even though I warmed it up. My gentle hand on their abdomen to palpate the liver and spleen was an irritant and made them giggle and jump off the examining table. They noticed everything.

"As time went on, I started to incorporate nutritional testing and discovered that every single hyperactive child I saw had low levels of calcium and magnesium. I became interested in controlling behavior with diet after I noticed how my daughter responded to foods. If she ate sugary stuff she'd have trouble, but if she ate complex carbohydrates or protein, her level of activity was fairly even. I found that hyperactive children did well when eating five small good meals a day.

"I was hoping to discover a sugar causation and not a hurt to the nervous system. I found that about 15 percent of these children did have some hurt to the nervous system, but that most of them came from family backgrounds of alcoholism, diabetes, and obesity, all sugar problems. I thought, 'Aha, I've got an answer here for hyperactivity. We should just stop the sugar.' It worked in a few cases, but not all.

"Then I saw that most of these children had had ear infections as infants. We know that ear infections in general indicate food sensitivity, usually to dairy products. I discovered that their present diets were usually laced with milk, cheese, ice cream, and lots of other dairy foods. Stopping all dairy helped some of these hyperactive children but it still wasn't the whole answer. It showed that some of these children had trouble absorbing calcium from dairy products because they were allergic to them. Almost all these children had circles under their eyes and had had their tonsils taken out. They had retracted eardrums and would constantly clear their throats. That indicated a sensitivity to dairy products. Their intestinal tracts prevented the uptake of calcium from the milk they were drinking. Their blood and hair levels of calcium and magnesium were very low. Also, they weren't getting the calcium and magnesium they needed. We all know that calcium and magnesium have a calming effect on people.

"After many years of investigation, I had learned that hyperactive children are often ticklish, goosey, and sensitive. They come from a family that has diabetes, obesity, or alcoholism. Generally, they're boys. Their teachers say they're in trouble. An especially important point is that they are usually okay one to one with their mother or father at home alone, but in a class of 30 other kids they cannot function. These children do better in small groups or one-on-one situations. That is ideal for them.

"Drug therapy helps them disregard unimportant stimuli. I found I could produce the same effect in most hyperactive children by giving them the right dose of calcium, usually 100 mg a day, and the right dose of magnesium, usually 500 mg a day. After receiving these minerals, usually 60 to 80 percent could manage without drug medication. It all seemed to fit. There was good evidence to indicate that hyperactive syndrome is related to food allergies, sensitivity to sugar, and not having enough calcium and magnesium.

"The next thing I noticed was that parents and teachers would report that many of these children were off and on, like Jekyll and Hyde. The parents would latch on to that little phrase as being almost diagnostic. That to me meant that it was not a psychiatric condition but a blood sugar fluctuation. It could come from eating sugar or from eating foods to which they were sensitive. We know that if people are sensitive to dairy products, for instance, the blood sugar will rise and get up to maybe 180 mg after eating a dairy food and then drop precipitously down to 60 mg. Then they crave these same dairy products again. They go up and down, up and down.

"If a teacher reports that a child is fine on Monday morning, doing his work and sitting still and then for no good reason on Monday afternoon he is all over the place, falling asleep or being disruptive, we can have a good idea that his behavior is related to something he ate for lunch. We have to carefully monitor the meals he eats and make sure the child doesn't get any particular food he is sensitive to. Along with milk the usual offenders are corn, wheat, soy, and eggs.

"The diet we recommend incorporates good foods as much as possible. Too much fruit may be detrimental due to the sugar. We recommend whole grain foods. We eliminate white bread, white rice, and empty-calorie foods. We don't have candy bars around. We don't have white soda crackers. We don't offer desserts to these children. We suggest good foods, complex carbohydrates, and vegetables, cooked as little as possible. Nibble, nibble, nibble is the rule we emphasize for hyperactive children. The whole family has to change their way of eating. Many of the parents find that they feel better on this diet as well.

"Once people change the diet of the hyperactive children, they find they can get off drugs, the Ritalin, Dexedrine, or whatever else they are on, or reduce the dosage, or take it only on tough exam days. My results showed that 80 percent of these hyperactive children were made 60 to 100 percent better. Most of the children and their parents would notice a change for the better but still feel that something was missing.

"Then I found, as I got more into a nutritional approach, that I needed to incorporate more vitamins. I was missing vitamin B$_6$, pyridoxine. I found that 50–100 mg of pyridoxine was very helpful, especially if the child had trouble with dream recall. This is also good for children who can't seem to concentrate.

"So there were two clues I looked for. I would ask teachers or parents of these children, 'Is he goosey, ticklish, sensitive?' If they were, I would know it had something to do with calcium and magnesium. If they said, 'He has a Jekyll-and-Hyde personality. He's on and off, good and bad,' then I knew the problem was related to diet. As I became more nutritionally aware, I found out that many of these children had trouble with their intestinal tracts. I gave them vitamin shots. They sting. If it really stung and really made them hyper, that was because they weren't absorbing enough calcium. That was another clue. If you have enough calcium in your muscles then the stingy shots aren't so painful.

"Many parents said the vitamin shots were very important and that they really made a difference to the child, but I had no way to figure out how much B_{12} and B_6 to give. It was helpful to me to find out that that could make some difference.

"In the past ten years I have been working with a chemist from Spokane named John Kitkoski who has discovered that most people in North America are somewhat alkaline. This may be the key as to why this condition had become more common in the past couple of decades. The earth is aging and has become more alkaline. The increased incidence of this condition, even though obstetrical management has gotten better, is because our foods have gotten worse and more processed.

"This alkalinity, from which many of us are suffering, is often the key to this problem. If people are somewhat alkaline, the minerals, like calcium and magnesium, are less soluble. It's more difficult for the minerals to work with the enzymes to do all the things that they're supposed to do for the body if the minerals—especially the calcium and the magnesium—are not soluble enough to be usable.

"This is the way we figure out whether someone is alkaline: When we evaluate the blood test, we add the levels of sodium and potassium in the blood, the alkaline elements, and we get a certain sum from that. Then we add the CO_2 and the chloride; these are acidic elements. That sum we subtract from the sum of the sodium and potassium. We should get a value between 6 and

12. Most people are above 12. This accounts for aches and pains, a narrow face, crowded teeth, certain allergies, a spastic colon, trouble absorbing foods. They could be eating the best food in the world, but if they're somewhat alkaline the nutrients in the food may not be available to them.

"This is why many people have found that becoming vegetarian has made a difference for them. Vegetarianism tends to make people more acidic because vinegar is produced. Most vegetarians don't have trouble with high blood pressure.

"We can sometimes spot these people. Say a child of nine or ten is somewhat hyperactive. He has circles under his eyes and he's got a nose full of junk. He's got a nasal sound. We look at his jaw and it's narrow. His front teeth are crowded. We know that this child probably was not breast fed and that he probably is alkaline and probably drinking cow's milk, to which he is sensitive. Therefore, he's not getting the calcium/magnesium he needs. He's probably craving calcium and magnesium because he knows somehow that he needs it. He doesn't know, however, that he won't be able to absorb it.

"It's been pointed out that most prisoners drink five times the amount of milk that ordinary people do. It may be the same phenomenon. They're looking for the calcium that they cannot absorb although their bodies are telling them they need this.

"So often at bottom it's a whole bunch of things causing the hyperactivity; it's never just one thing," Dr. Smith adds. "We were trained in medical school to make a diagnosis and to treat with a drug. The drug Ritalin is a standard for this. If it works that's a clue to me. If a stimulant has a calming effect then something is wrong with this person's ability to manufacture the right amount of norepinephrine for his limbic system. Therefore I can work on the diet and at the same time slow down the use of the Ritalin, which has side effects, such as leading to shortened stature. As this child grows up he is going to have to face the fact that he has got to change his diet."

Dr. Allan Spreen's approach to treating hyperactivity in both children and adults is very much in line with what we've been hearing from Dr. Smith. As Dr. Spreen states, "I have seen particularly hyperactive children who have an attention span of about two seconds. Often they are called autistic because they can't linger on any subject matter long enough to even begin to learn anything, much less give their parents a moment's peace. Often they are irritated by chemicals in their food that their system wasn't designed to handle: artificial color, artificial flavor, highly refined sugar, and flours and sugars that have had the nutrients required for their assimilation completely removed.

"My approach to hyperactivity is to try to get the individual biochemically in the best nutritional shape, and we usually get really nice results. Some people can have a very slightly sluggish thyroid that might not show up on blood tests. But with very low doses of thyroid, they feel so much better, even though their blood levels still remain normal on blood testing. Their whole emotional make-up improves. Their concentration gets better, and their energy level improves."

We conclude with a thought from Dr. Harold Buttram that should both worry us and at the same time remind us of how important it is that we continue to make our voices heard, so that the conventional medical establishment opens their ears and their hearts to the importance of nutrition in the treatment of illnesses with a mental component, in adults and in children: "I always make a point of asking patients of mine who are schoolteachers and have been teaching for 20 or 30 years whether there has been a change in the behavior of children during that time. The replies that I consistently receive are emphatic, that there has been a drastic change in children. There are more hyperactivity and attention deficit problems, more learning disorders, and more behavioral problems."

APPENDIX:
SCIENTIFIC ARTICLE SUMMARIES, BY
SUBJECT

The following are capsule descriptions of just some of the recent scientific articles that demonstrate the connection between nutritional factors and mental illness. The articles are all from respected peer-reviewed journals. They were assembled through a

231

computer search, then selected and edited at a cost of thousands of dollars to myself and my publisher.

Physicians reading this book will want to use this appendix as a matchless resource guide. It will lead them to the original scientific research, which in turn will bolster and substantiate the ideas and clinical strategies expounded in this book. I encourage you to follow this lead and have your secretary or assistant request reprints of individual articles that address your area of specialization directly from the medical journals themselves. You may find yourself more open to the practice of orthomolecular psychiatry than you ever expected.

For the general reader, you too will find that just reading the short summaries of some of the articles listed below will help strengthen your resolve. There is solid medical research to support many of the claims our contributing physicians have been making in earlier chapters.

AGGRESSION

A neuropsychopharmacological profile of "Cinkara," a polyherbal preparation. Sakina MR; Khan EA; Hamdard ME; Dandiya PC. Indian Journal of Physiology and Pharmacology, 1989 Jan–Mar, 33(1):43–6.

> In rats, the herbal preparation known as Cinkara appears to stimulate the central nervous system, but, unlike other such stimulants, it lowers aggressive behavior.

Acute and chronic effects of ginseng saponins on maternal aggression in mice. Yoshimura H; Watanabe K; Ogawa N. European Journal of Pharmacology, 1988 Jun 10, 150(3):319–24.

> Ginseng root contains an ingredient that suppresses maternal aggression in mice, without impairing their movement abilities.

Aminergic studies and cerebrospinal fluid actions in suicide. Banki CM; Arato M; Kilts CD. Annals of the New York Academy of Sciences, 1986, 487:221–30.

Suicidal psychiatric patients were shown to have significantly lower levels of magnesium in their cerebrospinal fluid than did a control group.

Anxiolytic activity of Panax ginseng roots: an experimental study. Bhattacharya SK; Mitra SK. Journal of Ethnopharmacology, 1991 Aug, 34(1):87–92.

Ginseng root was shown to be effective in reducing anxiety and aggression in rats and mice, when given over a period of 5 days (as opposed to single-dose administration, which had little effect). Ginseng's effectiveness was comparable to that of diazepam (Valium).

Cerebrospinal fluid magnesium and calcium related to amine metabolites, diagnosis, and suicide attempts. Banki CM; Vojnik M; Papp Z; Balla KZ; Arato M. Biological Psychiatry, 1985 Feb, 20(2):163–71.

Suicidal female psychiatric patients suffering from depression, schizophrenia, or adjustment disorder had decreased levels of magnesium in their cerebrospinal fluid.

Lithium in scalp hair of adults, students, and violent criminals. Effects of supplementation and evidence for interactions of lithium with vitamin B_{12} and with other trace elements. Schrauzer GN; Shrestha KP; Flores-Arce MF. Biological Trace Element Research, 1992 Aug, 34(2):161–76.

Lithium levels in human hair are low in certain pathological conditions, such as heart disease, and in learning disabled subjects and violent criminals. Hair levels of lithium rise with extradietary supplementation, and it is suggested that lithium may help distribute vitamin B_{12} in the body. Lithium also interacts with other trace elements.

Magnesium alters the potency of cocaine and haloperidol on mouse aggression. Kantak KM Psychopharmacology, 1989, 99(2):181–8.

Magnesium given to mice was shown to increase the

potency of a single dose of cocaine, and a magnesium-deficient diet reduced its potency. With chronic cocaine use, however, magnesium countered cocaine's effects.

Psychotropic effects of ginseng saponins on agonistic behavior between resident and intruder mice. Yoshimura H; Watanabe K; Ogawa N. European Journal of Pharmacology, 1988 Feb 9, 146(2–3):291–7.

Crude ginseng saponins and pure ginsenocide given to mice reduce aggressive behavior in certain situations.

Stimulant-like effects of magnesium on aggression in mice. Izenwasser SE; Garcia-Valdez K; Kantak KM. Pharmacology, Biochemistry and Behavior, 1986 Dec, 25(6):1195–9.

Low levels of magnesium in mice are linked to reduced aggression, heightened levels to increased aggression, and extremely high levels to reduced aggression. Since magnesium works with the neurotransmitters dopamine, norepinephrine, and serotonin, which affect aggressive behavior, the effects shown may be related to these systems.

ALCOHOLISM

A hypothetical mechanism for fetal alcohol syndrome involving ethanol inhibition of retinoic acid synthesis at the alcohol dehydrogenase step. Duester G. Alcoholism, Clinical and Experimental Research, 1991 Jun, 15(3):568–72.

A mechanism is offered to explain how ethanol causes the bodily abnormalities of fetal alcohol syndrome. To develop normally, embryonic tissues require certain levels of retinoic acid—the active form of vitamin A—and ethanol inhibits the enzyme needed to create this essential molecule.

ABC of Nutrition: Nutritional advice for other chronic diseases. Truswell, AS. Brit Med J. London: British Medical Association. July 20, 1985, v. 291, 197–200.

Nutritional guidelines are given for preventing various chronic diseases, including cirrhosis of the liver due to alcoholism.

Abnormalities of peripheral nerve conduction in relation to thiamine status in alcoholic patients. D'Amour ML; Bruneau J; Butterworth RF. Canadian Journal of Neurological Sciences, 1991 May, 18(2):126–8.

> Alcoholic patients were shown to be severely thiamine-deficient, a condition that may contribute to the nervous-system abnormalities seen in alcoholics. (Other factors that may be involved in these abnormalities are deficiencies of other vitamins, as well as the direct effects of alcohol itself.)

Age-related effects of chronic ethanol intake on vitamin A status in Fisher 344 rats. Mobarhan S; Seitz HK; Russell RM; Mehta R, Hupert J; Friedman H; Layden TJ; Meydani M; Langenberg P. Journal of Nutrition, 1991 Apr, 121(4):510–7.

> In rats, chronic ethanol ingestion alters tissue distribution of vitamin A.

Alcohol and bone disease. Rico H. Alcohol and Alcoholism, 1990, 25(4):345–52.

> Excessive alcohol consumption leads to decreased bone formation, defective mineralization, and osteoporosis, the latter due possibly to excessive zinc excretion induced by alcohol.

Alcohol, liver, and nutrition. Lieber CS. Journal of the American College of Nutrition, 1991 Dec, 10(6):602–32.

> Liver disease in alcoholics used to be attributed mainly to dietary deficiencies, but now more is understood about how alcohol affects the liver directly. It's been shown, for instance, that animals given ethanol, along with vitamin-A-rich diets, had low levels of the vitamin in their livers, and this was especially so when the ethanol was combined with other drugs, mimicking a common

circumstance in humans. When supplementing patients with vitamin A, however, it is essential to understand that too much of the vitamin is toxic to the liver—and that this is particularly so in alcoholics—so that the amount given is crucial. This decreased "therapeutic window" for alcoholics taking vitamin A applies to other nutritional supplements as well.

Alcohol-induced bone marrow damage: status before and after a 4-week period of abstinence from alcohol with or without disulfiram. A randomized bone marrow study in alcohol-dependent individuals. Casagrande G; Michot F. Blut, 1989 Sep, 59(3):231–6.

Alcohol can induce bone marrow damage, which has been shown to be reversed in patients who totally abstain. However, patients who detoxified while taking the drug disulfiram (Antabuse) continued to have bone marrow pathology.

Alcoholism in the elderly. How to spot and treat a problem the patient wants to hide. Tobias CR: Lippmann S; Pary R; Oropilla T; Embry CK. Postgraduate Medicine, 1989 Sep 15, 86(4):67–70, 75–9.

Increased awareness of alcoholism by physicians, with early diagnosis and treatment, can reduce its damaging effects. Especially in the elderly, all medications used should be monitored, and nonessential ones should be discontinued. Also suggested are treating withdrawal symptoms with thiamine, multivitamins, and perhaps sedatives; treating any underlying psychiatric disorder; psychosocial support; and possibly the use of disulfiram (Antabuse).

Anemia in alcoholics. Savage D; Lindenbaum J. Medicine, 1986 Sep, 65(5):322–38.

A deficiency of folic acid in alcoholics is a factor in anemia in these patients. A diagnostic approach to anemia in alcoholics was developed, as were suggestions for therapy.

Ascorbic acid chronic alcohol consumption in the guinea pig. Susick RL Jr; Abrams GD; Zurawski CA; Zannoni VG. Toxicology and Applied Pharmacology, 1986 Jun 30, 84(2):329–35.

> Protection against the toxic effects of chronic alcohol consumption was observed in guinea pigs maintained on a high-ascorbic-acid diet, as opposed to those on a low-ascorbic-acid diet.

Assessment of nutritional status and in vivo immune responses in a disease. Mills PR; Shenkin A; Anthony, RS; McLelland, AS; Alistair NH; MacSween RNM; Russell RI. Am. J. Clin. Nutr., Bethesda, Md.: American Society for Clinical Nutrition 1983. v.38(6)p.849–859.

> High alcohol intake resulted in metabolic and cellular changes, including the depletion of potassium, magnesium, and phosphate in the blood.

Blood thiamine and thiamine phosphate concentrations in excessive drinkers with or without peripheral neuropathy. Poupon RF; Gervaise G; Riant P; Houin G; Tillement JP. Alcohol and Alcoholism, 1990, 25(6):605–11.

> Thiamine phosphate (but not free thiamine) was found to be at low levels in groups of excessive drinkers with and without peripheral nerve damage.

Bone and mineral metabolism and chronic alcohol abuse. Lalor BC; France MW; Powell D; Adams PH; Counihan TB. Quarterly Journal of Medicine, 1986 May, 59(229):497–511.

> Significant changes in bone structure and mass appear to be common among heavy drinkers. In a group of alcoholic patients with varying degrees of liver damage, but with no clinical evidence of metabolic bone disease, osteoporosis and osteomalacia were found, and related to various factors, including magnesium deficiency, low blood levels of calcitriol, the state of liver function, and the type of alcohol consumed.

Calcium status and calcium-regulating hormones in alcoholics. Bjorneboe GE; Bjorneboe A. Johnsen J; Skylv N; Oftebro H; Gautvik KM; Hoiseth A; Morland J; Drevon CA. Alcoholism, Clinical and Experimental Research, 1988 Apr, 12(2):229–32.

> Vitamin D_3 levels were shown to be lower in alcoholics than in a control group, during the winter season. Dietary intake of the vitamin did not differ significantly between the groups, and so it seems that the activities of enzymes crucial in vitamin D_3 metabolism may be altered in alcoholics, resulting in low calcium levels.

Carotenoids and liposoluble vitamins in liver cirrhosis. Rocchi E; Borghi A; Paolillo F; Pradelli M; Casalgrandi G. Journal of Laboratory and Clinical Medicine, 1991 Aug, 118(2):176–85.

> The role of carotenoids, retinol, and tocopherol in quenching oxidative cellular damage and combatting tumor growth is well documented; this research looked at their activity in human liver cirrhosis. In patients with this disease, significantly reduced blood levels were found of alpha- and beta-carotene and several other vitamin factors. Improved diet for patients with liver cirrhosis is discussed.

Changes in the activation of red blood cell transketolase of alcoholic patients during treatment. Jeyasingham MD; Pratt OE; Shaw GK; Thomson AD. Alcohol and Alcoholism, 1987, 22(4):359–65.

> An enzyme test can monitor the effectiveness of thiamin therapy used in alcohol detoxification.

Chronic administration of ethanol with high vitamin A supplementation in a liquid diet to rats does not cause liver fibrosis. 1. Morphological observations. Bosma A; Seifert WF; Wilson JH; Roholl PJ; Brouwer A; Knook DL. Journal of Hepatology, 1991 Sep, 13(2):240–8.

> Rats fed a high-ethanol diet supplemented with vitamin A did not develop liver fibrosis, suggesting that the main effects of chronic ethanol consumption to the liver may

be secondary to interference with host resistance to infections.

Chronic administration of ethanol with high vitamin A supplementation in a liquid diet to rats does not cause liver fibrosis. 2. Biochemical observations. Seifert WF; Bosma A; Hendriks HF; Blaner WS; van Leeuwen RE; van Thiel-de Ruiter GC; Wilson JH; Knook DL; Brouwer A. Journal of Hepatology, 1991 Sep, 13(2):249–55.

> The inability of a high-alcohol, high-vitamin-A diet to induce liver fibrosis in rats (see abstract above) was further evaluated. The hypothesis that interaction between alcohol and retinoids is a major factor in alcoholic liver disease needs to be reconsidered.

Chronic alcohol treatment results in disturbed vitamin D metabolism and skeletal abnormalities in rats. Turner RT; Aloia RC; Sogol LD; Hannon KS; Bell NH. Alcoholism, Clinical and Experimental Research, 1988 Feb, 12(1):159–62.

> Rats on a high-alcohol diet, when compared to a control group, had low blood levels of magnesium and of substances metabolized from vitamin D.

Chronic ethanol feeding and acute ethanol exposure in vitro: effect on intestinal transport of biotin. Said HM; Sharifian A; Bagherzadeh A; Mock D. American Journal of Clinical Nutrition, 1990 Dec, 52(6):1083–6.

> Alcohol-fed rats showed lowered biotin levels in their blood, as well as lowered ability to absorb biotin from the intestine.

Concentrations of zinc and copper in pregnant problem drinkers and infants. Halmesmaki E; Ylikorkala, O; Alfthan G. Brit. Med. J. London: British Medical Association. Nov 23, 1985. v. 291, 1470–1471.

> Reduced zinc levels were found in infants of mothers who were problem drinkers.

Current progress toward the prevention of the Wernicke-Korsakoff syndrome. Bishai DM; Bozzetti LP. Alcohol and Alcoholism, 1986, 21(4):315–23.

> Wernicke-Korsakoff syndrome, a neurological disorder seen mainly in alcoholics, may be prevented by supplementing alcoholic beverages with thiamin. Also relevant to the disease are folate and magnesium levels.

Decreased serum selenium in alcoholics as related to liver structure and function. Korpela H; Kumpulainen J; Luoma PV; Arranto AJ. Am. J. Clin. Nutr., Bethesda, Md.: American Society for Clinical Nutrition 1985. v. 42(1):147–151.

> A group of alcoholic patients showed low blood levels of selenium, with those patients having the most damaged livers showing the lowest levels. Inadequate dietary selenium intake, as well as alcohol-caused changes in liver structure and function, are probable factors.

Depressed selenium and vitamin E levels in an alcoholic population. Possible relationship to hepatic injury through increased lipid peroxidation. Tanner AR; Bantock I; Hinks L; Lloyd B; Turner NR; Wright R. Digestive Diseases and Sciences, 1986 Dec, 31(12):1307–12.

> Blood levels of both selenium and vitamin E were shown to be significantly depressed in alcoholics, with selenium more markedly depressed in those with established liver disease. Depressed selenium correlated closely with poor nutritional status, and liver disease activity was more markedly abnormal in subjects with combined vitamin E and selenium deficiency.

Diminished serum concentration of vitamin E in alcoholics. Bjorneboe GE; Johnsen J; Bjorneboe A; Bache-Wiig JE; Morland J; Drevon CA. *Annals of Nutrition and Metabolism*, 1988, 32(2):56–61.

> A group of alcoholic subjects showed low blood levels of vitamin E when compared with a control group, and it

was reported as well that their estimated dietary intake of this vitamin was significantly lower than that of the controls. Selenium was also lower in the alcoholics, and the reduced levels of these substances may affect cell structure and function, and contribute to development of diseases frequently observed in alcoholics.

Discovery and importance of zinc in human nutrition. Prasad AS. *Fed. Proc. Fed. Am. Soc. Exp. Biol.*, Bethesda, Md.: The Federation. Oct 1984. (13):2829–2834.

Zinc appears to be involved in many biological functions; its roles in enzymatic functions, cell membranes, and immunity have been well established. Cases of deficiency of this trace element can be traced to several causes, and alcoholism is a predisposing factor.

Disorders of divalent ions and vitamin D metabolism in chronic alcoholism. Pitts TO; Van Thiel DH. *Recent Developments in Alcoholism*, 1986, 4:357–77.

Deficient vitamin D metabolism in alcoholics can result from liver problems, lack of sun exposure, poor diet, and malabsorption. Low vitamin D may contribute to calcium and phosphate deficiencies, and to osteoporosis. Alcoholics should be screened for vitamin D deficiency and given supplements if needed.

Effect of abstinence from alcohol on the depressin of glutathione peroxidase activity and selenium and vitamin E levels in chronic alcoholic patients. Girre C; Hispard E; Therond P; Guedj S.; Bourdon R; Dally S. *Alcoholism, Clinical and Experimental Research*, 1990 Dec, 14(6):909–12.

Chronic alcoholics without severe liver disease were shown to have deficiencies in their antioxidant defense systems. Blood factors indicating this were seen to normalize during 14 days of alcohol abstinence.

Effect of alcohol consumption on serum concentration of 25-hydroxyvitamin D_3, retinol, and retinol-binding protein.

Bjorneboe GE; Johnsen J; Bjorneboe A; Rousseau B; Pederson JI; Norum KR; Morland J; Drevon CA. *American Journal of Clinical Nutrition*, 1986 Nov, 44(5):678–82.

Chronic alcohol consumers had significantly lower levels of vitamin D in their blood than did a control group, even though the two groups seemed to have similar dietary intake of the nutrient. The alcoholics also had lower calcium levels.

Effect of chronic consumption of ethanol and vitamin E on fatty acid composition and lipid peroxidation in rat heart tissue. Pirozhkov SV; Eskelson CD; Watson RR; Hunter GC; Piotrowski JJ; Bernhard V. *Alcohol*, 1992 Jul–Aug, 9(4):329–34.

Rats were given large amounts of ethanol and vitamin E, and the latter was shown to have a stabilizing effect on phospholipids in the heart, by preventing their deterioration.

Effect of chronic ethanol administration on thiamine transport in microvillous vesicles of rat small intestine. Gastaldi G; Casirola D; Ferrari G; Rindi G. *Alcohol and Alcoholism*, 1989, 24(2):83–9.

Intestinal absorption of thiamine was markedly lower in rats that had been administered ethanol over a period of time than in nonalcoholic rats.

Effect of free radical scavengers on superoxide dismutase (SOD) enzyme in patients with alcoholic cirrhosis. Feher J; Lang I; Nekam K; Muzes G; Deak G. *Acta Medica Hungarica*, 1988, 45(3–4):265–76.

Silymarin and other antioxidants have an effect protective of the liver in alcoholics.

Effect of heavy alcohol consumption on serum concentrations of fat-soluble vitamins and selenium. Bjorneboe GA; Johnsen J; Bjorneboe A; Morland J; Drevon CA. *Alcohol and Alcoholism*, 1987, Suppl 1:533–7.

A group of alcoholics showed blood levels of vitamin E

and selenium that were significantly lower than those of a control group, and it is noted that these antioxidants protect against cell damage. Also lower in the alcoholics was vitamin D; this may be a factor—through disturbance of calcium and phosphate metabolism—in the high frequency of bone fractures and osteomalacia in alcoholics.

Effect of silibinin on the activity and expression of superoxide dismutase in lymphocytes from patients with chronic alcoholic liver disease. Feher J; Lang I; Nekam K; Csomos G; Muzes G; Deak G. *Free Radical Research Communications*, 1987, 3(6):373–7.

Silibinin acts to protect the liver, possibly through antioxidant activity.

Effects of acute ethanol on urinary excretion of 5-methyltetrahydrofolic acid and folate derivatives in the rat. Eisenga BH; Collins TD; McMartin KE. *Journal of Nutrition*, 1989 Oct, 119(10):1498–505.

Ethanol-treated rats were shown to excrete more folic acid in their urine than did a control group. This effect has been implicated in the deficiency of this vitamin often seen in alcoholics.

Ethanol and fetal nutrition: effect of chronic ethanol exposure on rat placental growth and membrane-associated folic acid receptor binding activity. Fisher SE; Inselman LS; Duffy L; Atkinson M; Spencer H; Chang B. *Journal of Pediatric Gastroenterology and Nutrition*, 1985 Aug, 4(4):645–9.

Rat fetuses whose mothers were fed alcohol were smaller than those of control-group mothers, and their placentas were less able to process folic acid.

Folate absorption in alcoholic pigs: in vitro hydrolysis and transport at the intestinal brush border membrane. Naughton CA; Chandler CJ; Duplantier RB; Halsted CH. *American Journal of Clinical Nutrition*, 1989 Dec, 50(6):1436–41.

An enzymatic process required for intestinal absorption of folic acid was seen, in the miniature pig, to be impeded by chronic consumption of alcohol.

Food and nutrient intake of alcoholic laborers. Chhabra KB; Ramesh P; Mehta U. *Ecol. Food Nutr. London*: Gordon & Breach Science Publishers. 1991. v.2, 51–57.

Fifty subjects—30 alcoholics and 20 nonalcoholics— were selected from an industrial area of Ludhiana City, Punjab, India, and their dietary intake was assessed. Although both groups consumed about the same number of calories, the nutrient intake of the alcoholics was lower, resulting in deficiencies.

Hypothesis: prenatal ethanol-induced birth defects and retinoic acid. Pullarkat RK. *Alcoholism, Clinical and Experimental Research*, 1991 Jun, 15(3):565–7.

Prenatal exposure to alcohol causes birth defects in humans and animals, specifically, central nervous system and limb abnormalities. It is hypothesized that this comes about as a result of ethanol's inhibitory effect of the formation of retinoic acid from retinol. Retinoic acid is important in the development of the central nervous system, and of limbs.

Inhibitory effect of maternal alcohol ingestion on rat pup hepatic 25-hydroxyvitamin D production. Milne M; Baran DT. *Pediatric Research*, 1985 Jan, 19(1):102–4.

Eighteen days of alcohol consumption had no effect on liver synthesis of vitamin D in pregnant rats, but did inhibit fetal production of the vitamin.

Interaction of alcohol with other drugs and nutrients. Implication for the therapy of alcoholic liver disease. Lieber CS. *Drugs*, 1990, 40 Suppl 3:23–44.

New understanding of how alcohol damages the liver has led to more successful therapy with drugs and nutritional factors, such as vitamin A. Vitamin A is depleted in the alcoholic, but excess vitamin A is extra-toxic in the alcoholic.

Interaction of niacin and zinc metabolism in patients with alcoholic pellagra. Vannucchi H; Moreno FS. *American Journal of Clinical Nutrition*, 1989 Aug, 50(2):364–9.

> In patients with alcoholic pellagra, zinc interacts with niacin metabolism, through a probable mediation by vitamin B_6.

Intestinal absorption, liver uptake, and excretion of 3H-folic acid in folic acid-deficient, alcohol-consuming nonhuman primates. Blocker DE; Thenen SW. *American Journal of Clinical Nutrition*, 1987 Sep, 46(3):503–10.

> Chronic alcohol ingestion in nonhuman primates impaired folic acid utilization.

Iron uptake from transferrin and asialotransferrin by hepatocytes from chronically alcohol-fed rats. Potter BJ; McHugh TA; Beloqui O. *Alcoholism, Clinical and Experimental Research*, 1992 Aug, 16(4):810–5.

> Alcohol-fed rats showed impaired ability to use iron.

Lipoprotein cholesterol, vitamin A, and vitamin E in an alcoholic population. D'Antonio JA; LaPorte RE; Dai WS; Hom DL; Wozniczak M; Kuller LH. *Cancer*, 1986 May 1, 57(9):1798–802.

> Elevated alcohol consumption is associated with increased cancer risk, due possibly to altered vitamin A, vitamin E, and cholesterol metabolism in alcoholics.

Liver cell protection in toxic liver lesion. Feher J; Cornides A; Pal J; Lang I; Csomos G. *Acta Physiologica Hungarica*, 1989, 73(2–3):285–91.

> In animal experiments, silymarin, silibinin, and Aica-P were shown to have liver-protecting effects related to their actions as free-radical scavengers.

Metabolism of vitamin D in patients with primary biliary cirrhosis and alcoholic liver disease. Mawer EB; Klass HJ; Warnes TW; Berry JL. *Clinical Science*, 1985 Nov, 69(5):561–70.

Alchoholism may lead to impairment of the liver's function in processing vitamin D.

Nutrition and alcoholic encephalopathies. Thomson AD; Jeyasingham MD; Pratt OE; Shaw GK. *Acta Medica Scandinavica*. Supplementum, 1987, 717:55–65.

Chronic alcoholism may cause vitamin B deficiencies due to impaired uptake of thiamin as well as disruption of thiamin metabolism. This may subsequently cause brain damage.

Plasma amino acid patterns in alcoholic pellagra patients. Vannucchi H; Moreno FS; Amarante AR; de Oliveira JE; Marchini JS. *Alcohol and Alcoholism*, 1991, 26(4):431–6.

Alcoholics with pellagra (a disease resulting from lack of B complex vitamins) showed lowered levels for 11 amino acids in the blood.

Plasma osteocalcin levels in liver cirrhosis. Capra F; Casaril M; Gabrielli GB; Stanzial A; Ferrari S; Gandini G; Falezza G; Corrocher R. *Italian Journal of Gastroenterology*, 1991 Mar–Apr, 23(3):124–7.

Cirrhosis of the liver results in lowered levels of osteocalcin, and therefore a lowered ability to replace bone. The low osteocalcin levels may be due to low vitamin D and blood calcium levels.

Prenatal ethanol exposure decreases hippocampal mossy fiber zinc in 45-day-old rats. Savage DD; Montano CY; Paxton LL; Kasarskis EJ. *Alcoholism, Clinical and Experimental Research*, 1989 Aug, 13(4):588–93.

In rats, a brain region important in the process of memory consolidation is affected by prenatal exposure to alcohol. Pregnant rats on an alcohol diet had offspring with lower than normal zinc levels in the hippocampal formation.

Randomized controlled trial of silymarin treatment in patients with cirrhosis of the liver. Ferenci P; Dragosics B; Dittrich H; Frank H; Benda L; Lochs H; Meryn S; Base W; Schneider B. *Journal of Hepatology*, 1989 Jul, 9(1):105–13.

> Silymarin, the active principle of the milk thistle, Silybum marianum, protects experimental animals against various substances toxic to the liver. In a double-blind study of human patients with cirrhosis, silymarin was shown to have an effect protective of the liver.

Reduced concentration of hepatic alpha-tocopherol in patients with alcoholic liver cirrhosis. Bell H; Bjorneboe A; Eidsvoll B; Norum KR; Raknerud N; Try K; Thomassen Y; Drevon CA. *Alcohol and Alcoholism*, 1992 Jan, 27(1):39–46.

> The vitamin E content in the liver was significantly lower in patients with alcoholic cirrhosis compared with patients with normal livers.

Role of acetyl-L-carnitine in the treatment of cognitive deficit in chronic alcoholism. Tempesta E; Troncon R; Janiri L; Colusso L; Riscica P; Saraceni G; Gesmundo E; Calvani M; Benedetti N; Pola P. *International Journal of Clinical Pharmacology Research*, 1990, 10(1–2):101–7.

> Acetyl-L-carnitine can be a useful and safe therapeutic agent in ameliorating the cognitive disturbances of chronic alcoholics. Fifty-five one-month-abstinent alcoholics were put in a double-blind placebo-controlled study to assess the effects of the substance, which did help the group that took it perform better or regain performance abilities faster than those who did not. Memory, logic, and constructional abilities were among those improved.

Selenium status in patients with liver cirrhosis and alcoholism. Johansson U; Johnsson F; Joelsson B; Berglund M; Akesson B. *British Journal of Nutrition*, 1986 Mar, 55(2):227–33.

Blood levels of selenium and vitamins A and E were shown to be reduced in patients with alcoholic cirrhosis.

Some aspects of antioxidant status in blood from alcoholics. Bjorneboe GE; Johnsen J; Bjorneboe A; Marklund SL; Skylv N; Hoiseth A; Bache-Wiig JE; Morland J; Drevon CA. *Alcoholism, Clinical and Experimental Research*, 1988 Dec, 12(6):806–10.

Blood levels of vitamin E were 30 percent lower in a group of alcoholics compared to a control group of nonalcoholics. After this measurement was taken, half of the alcoholics in the study received vitamin E supplementation, as did half of the nonalcoholics; the other halves of each group were supplemented with placebo capsules. Of the four groups, only the alcoholics receiving the vitamin E supplements showed increased blood levels of the vitamin, showing that reduced levels of vitamin E can be normalized by supplementation.

The Wernicke-Korsakoff syndrome in Queensland, Australia: antecedents and prevention. Price J. *Alcohol and Alcoholism*, 1985, 20(2):233–42.

Wernicke-Korsakoff syndrome may be the end result of thiamine deficiency in alcoholics. To prevent the syndrome, fortification of alcoholic beverages with thiamine has been proposed in Queensland, Australia, and the publicity this suggestion has generated has alerted some heavy drinkers to the need for supplementary B vitamins.

The antioxidant status of patients with either alcohol-induced liver damage or myopathy. Ward RJ; Peters TJ. *Alcohol and Alcoholism*, 1992 Jul, 27(4):359–65.

Alcoholics showed low blood levels of beta-carotene, zinc, and selenium, and in patients with alcoholic cirrhosis, alpha-tocopherol levels were also low.

The clinical spectrum of alcoholic pellagra encephalopathy. A retrospective analysis of 22 cases studied pathologically. Serdaru

M; Hausser-Hauw C; Laplane D; Buge A; Castaigne P; Goulon M; Lhermitte F; Hauw JJ. *Brain*, 1988 Aug, 111 (Pt 4):829–42.

Alcoholic pellagra has often gone unrecognized, and therefore untreated with niacin. Multiple vitamin therapy should be given in the treatment of undiagnosed brain abnormalities in alcoholic patients.

The concentration of thiamin and thiamin phosphate esters in patients with alcoholic liver cirrhosis. Tallaksen CM; Bell H; Bohmer T. *Alcohol and Alcoholism*, 1992 Sep, 27(5):523–30.

Current alcohol misuse was shown to be associated with low thiamin concentrations in the blood.

The effect of vitamin E (alpha-tocopherol) supplementation on hepatic levels of vitamin A and E in ethanol and cod liver oil fed rats. Odeleye OE; Eskelson CD; Alak JI; Watson RR; Chvapil M; Mufti SI; Earnest D. *International Journal for Vitamin and Nutrition Research*, 1991, 61(2):143–8.

Ethanol consumption in rats resulted in decreased levels of vitamins A and E in their livers, but supplementation with vitamin E restored levels of this vitamin to normal, and restored levels of vitamin A somewhat. Rats consuming cod liver oil along with ethanol also had lowered vitamin A and E levels, although the levels were higher than those of the rats not receiving cod liver oil.

Thiamin deficiency and prevention of the Wernicke-Korsakoff syndrome. A major public health problem. Yellowlees PM. *Medical Journal of Australia*, 1986 Sep 1, 145(5):216–9.

In order to prevent Wernicke-Korsakoff syndrome in Australia, it is recommended that flour and bread, as well as alcoholic beverages, be fortified with thiamin.

Thiamin status and biochemical indices of malnutrition and alcoholism in settled communities of !Kung San. van der Westhuyzen J; Davis RE; Icke GC; Jenkins T. *Journal of Tropical Medicine and Hygiene*, 1987 Dec, 90(6):283–9.

Settled groups of !Kung San in the northern Kalahari Desert of Namibia show a high prevalence of thiamin deficiency, and alcohol abuse seems to be the main factor.

Tissue thiamin levels of hospitalised alcoholics before and after oral or parenteral vitamins. Baines M; Bligh JG; Madden JS. *Alcohol and Alcoholism*, 1988, 23(1):49–52.

Oral supplementation of thiamin is effective for most alcoholics.

Trace element and vitamin deficiency in alcoholic and control subjects. Cook CC; Walden RJ; Graham BR; Gillham C, Davies S; Prichard BN. *Alcohol and Alcoholism*, 1991, 26(5–6):541–8.

A wide range of trace elements and vitamins was studied in alcoholic patients admitted for detoxification and in healthy controls. The alcoholics were found to be deficient relative to the controls in magnesium and vitamin E, but there was also a surprising range of deficiencies in the control group, which points to the prevalence of undetected nutritional deficiency in the general population.

Vitamin A status of alcoholics upon admission and after two weeks of hospitalization. Chapman KM; Prabhudesai M; Erdman JW Jr. *Journal of the American College of Nutrition*, 1993 Feb, 12(1):77–83.

Elevated bilirubin levels seen in alcoholics may indicate low vitamin A levels. Caution in levels of vitamin A therapy in these cases is advised, and consideration should instead be given to beta-carotene supplementation.

Vitamin B_{12} and folate function in chronic alcoholic men with peripheral neuropathy and encephalopathy. Gimsing P; Melgaard B; Andersen K; Vilstrup H; Hippe E. *Journal of Nutrition*, 1989 Mar, 119(3):416–24.

Folate deficiency may contribute to the development of nerve problems in alcoholics.

Vitamin B$_6$ status in cirrhotic patients in relation to apoenzyme of serum alanine aminotransferase. Ohgi N; Hirayama C. *Clinical Biochemistry*, 1988 Dec, 21(6):367–70.

Alcoholic cirrhotic patients have vitamin B$_6$ deficiency.

Vitamin K deficiency in chronic alcoholic males. Iber FL; Shamszad M; Miller PA; Jacob R. *Alcoholism, Clinical and Experimental Research*, 1986 Dec, 10(6):679–81.

Blood clotting defects are frequently present in alcoholics, suggesting vitamin K deficiency. Alcoholics given vitamin K did show more normal clotting protein in their blood than those not given the vitamin.

Zinc and vitamin A status of alcoholics in a medical unit in Sri Lanka. Atukorala TM; Herath CA; Ramachandran S. *Alcohol and Alcoholism*, 1986, 21(3):269–75.

Alcoholics had lower blood levels of zinc and vitamin A than did controls, with female alcoholics having levels lower than those of males, although they drank less.

Zinc nutrition in fetal alcohol syndrome. Keppen LD; Moore DJ; Cannon DJ. *Neurotoxicology*, 1990 Summer, 11(2):375–80.

Experiments with mice suggest that zinc intake should be optimized during pregnancy; the Recommended Daily Allowance should not be exceeded.

ALZHEIMER'S DISEASE

A histochemical study of iron, transferrin, and ferritin in Alzheimer's diseased brains. Connor JR; Menzies SL; St. Martin SM; Mufson EJ. *Journal of Neuroscience Research*, 1992 Jan, 31(1):75–83.

Iron, and iron-regulating proteins, are abnormally distributed in the brains of Alzheimer's disease patients.

A natural and broad spectrum nootropic substance for treatment of SDAT—the Ginkgo biloba extract. Funfgeld EW. *Progress in Clinical and Biological Research*, 1989, 317:1247–60.

Ginkgo biloba extract was found to be therapeutic, and without side effects, in Parkinson's patients with additional signs of Alzheimer's-type dementia.

A search for longitudinal variations in trace element levels in nails of Alzheimer's disease patients. Vance DE; Ehmann WD; Markesbery WR. *Biological Trace Element Research*, 1990 Jul–Dec, 26–27:461–70.

Progressive changes in trace-element levels occur in the nails of Alzheimer's disease patients, and imbalances are detected even in the earliest stages of the disease. Mercury levels were seen to decrease progressively with the level of the disease and with age, and potassium and zinc to increase with these same factors.

Acetyl-L-carnitine: a drug able to slow the progress of Alzheimer's disease? Carta A; Calvani M. *Annals of the New York Academy of Sciences*, 1991, 640:228–32.

Clinical studies suggest that acetyl-L-carnitine, which has protective effects against aging processes and nerve degeneration, may slow the natural course of Alzheimer's disease.

Changes in calcium homeostasis during aging and Alzheimer's disease. Peterson C; Ratan R; Shelanski M; Goldman J. *Annals of the New York Academy of Sciences*, 1989, 568:262–70.

Alzheimer's disease patients and normal aged patients had altered calcium regulation compared to that of young patients.

Cultured cells as a screen for novel treatments of Alzheimer's disease. Malow BA; Baker AC; Blass JP. *Archives of Neurology*, 1989 Nov. 46(11):1201–3.

L-carnitine normalized two properties normally measured as abnormal in Alzheimer's diseased cells.

Double-blind parallel design pilot study of acetyl levocarnitine in patients with Alzheimer's disease. Sano M; Bell K; Cote L;

Dooneief G; Lawton A; Legler L; Marder K; Naini A; Stern Y; Mayeux R. *Archives of Neurology*, 1992 Nov, 49(11):1137–41.

Acetyl levocarnitine shows the ability to retard the deterioration in some cognitive areas in those suffering from Alzheimer's disease.

Effects of free Ca^{2+} on the $[Ca^{2+} + Mg^{2+}]$-dependent adenosinetriphosphatase (ATPase) of Alzheimer and normal fibroblasts. Rizopoulos E; Chambers JP; Wayner MJ; Martinez AO; Armstrong LS. *Neurobiology of Aging*, 1989 Nov–Dec, 10(6):717–20.

Calcium regulation is different in Alzheimer's disease cells than in normal cells.

Essential fatty acids in Alzheimer's disease. Corrigan FM; Van Rhijn A; Horrobin DF. *Annals of the New York Academy of Sciences*, 1991, 640:250–2.

Essential fatty acids are abnormal in Alzheimer's disease patients. Twenty-week treatment with essential fatty acids improved the levels.

Folate, vitamin B_{12} and cognitive impairment in patients with Alzheimer's disease. Levitt AJ; Karlinsky H. *Acta Psychiatrica Scandinavica*, 1992 Oct, 86(4):301–5.

An inverse relationship was found between vitamin B_{12} levels and the severity of cognitive impairment in Alzheimer's disease patients.

Hair aluminium in normal aged and senile dementia of Alzheimer type. Kobayashi S; Fujiwara S; Arimoto S; Koide H; Fukuda J; Shimode K; Yamaguchi S; Okada K; Tsunematsu T. *Progress in Clinical and Biological Research*, 1989, 317:1095–109.

In Alzheimer's disease, decreased calcium and magnesium levels enhance accumulation of aluminum in the brain. In normal aged individuals, cerebral blood flow levels decrease as hair aluminum levels increase, suggesting that aluminum may contribute to aging of the brain.

Hypothesis regarding amyloid and zinc in the pathogenesis of Alzheimer disease: potential for preventive intervention. Constantinidis, J. *Alzheimer Disease and Associated Disorders*, 1991 Spring, 5(1):31–5.

> It is suggested that amyloid production in the cerebral cortex causes a zinc deficiency in the brain; toxic metals (such as iron, aluminum, and mercury) then displace the zinc in some enzymes. Application of a zinc complex that crosses the blood-brain barrier may mitigate these effects.

Lipid peroxidation and free radical scavengers in Alzheimer's disease. Jeandel C; Nicolas MB; Dubois F; Nabet-Belleville F; Penin F; Cuny G. *Gerontology*, 1989, 35(5–6):275–82.

> The blood of a group of Alzheimer's patients, when compared with that of a group of healthy age-matched controls, showed lower levels of glutathione peroxidase activity in red blood cells, as well as lower levels of vitamins E, C, and A, and zinc.

Long-term acetyl-L-carnitine treatment in Alzheimer's disease. Spagnoli A; Lucca U; Menasce G; Bandera L; Cizza G; Forloni G; Tettamanti M; Frattura L; Tiraboschi P; Comelli M. *Neurology*, 1991 Nov, 41(11):1726–32.

> The effects of acetyl-L-carnitine on Alheimer's patients were assessed in a double-blind, placebo-controlled study over one year. After this period, both the treated and plcebo groups worsened, but the treated group showed a slower rate of deterioration in 13 of the 14 outcome measures, with statistically significant results in five of them. No significant side effects were seen.

Low B_{12} levels related to high activity of platelet MAO in patients with dementia disorders. A retrospective study. Regland B; Gottfries CG; Oreland L; Svennerholm L. *Acta Psychiatrica Scandinavica*, 1988 Oct, 78(4):451–7.

> Vitamin B_{12} levels were shown to be reduced in the blood

of Alzheimer's patients and patients with confusional states.

Magnesium depletion and pathogenesis of Alzheimer's disease. Durlach J. *Magnesium Research*, 1990 Sep, 3(3):217–8.

> Magnesium depletion in a particular region of the brain, along with aluminum incorporation into the brain, is associated with Alzheimer's disease. Further research should seek to control the alterations of albumin, which may induce the magnesium depletion.

Nutrient intakes and energy expenditures of residents with senile Alzheimer's type. Litchford MD; Wakefield LM. *J. Am. Diet Assoc.*, Chicago, Ill.: The Association, Feb 1987. v. 87(2).

> In a study conducted over three days, Alzheimer's patients were seen to exhibit lower nutrient intake than did a control group. Significant intake differences were noted for vitamin A, thiamin, niacin, riboflavin, and calcium, as well as for total calories and other factors.

Oxidative damage in Alzheimer's dementia, and the potential etiopathogenic role of aluminosilicates, microglia and micronutrient interactions. Evans PH; Yano E; Klinowski J; Peterhans E. *Exs*, 1992, 62:178–89.

> In laboratory experiments, aluminosilicate particles have stimulated the generation of tissue-damaging free radicals in nervous-system cells. Similar aluminosilicate deposits have been found in the brains of Alzheimer's patients, and it is suggested that antioxidant micronutrients and pharmacological agents would be useful in preventing and treating Alzheimer's disease.

Plasma concentrations of vitamins A and E and carotenoids in Alzheimer's disease. Zaman Z; Roche S; Fielden P; Frost PG; Niriella DC; Cayley AC. *Age and Ageing*, 1992 Mar, 21(2):91–4.

> Compared to controls, Alzheimer's patients had lower levels of vitamins E and A, and of beta-carotene, in their blood.

Possible participation of calcium-regulating factors in senile dementia in elderly female subjects. Ogihara T; Miya K; Morimoto S. *Gerontology*, 1990, 36 Suppl 1:25–30.

> Calcium and calcium-regulating hormones may play several roles in senile dementia.

Regional distribution of iron and iron-regulatory proteins in the brain in aging and Alzheimer's disease. Connor JR; Snyder BS; Beard JL; Fine RE; Mufson EJ. *Journal of Neuroscience Research*, 1992 Feb, 31(2):327–35.

> Levels of blood proteins that regulate the body's use of iron are altered in the aging brain, particularly in Alzheimer's disease. The decreased availability of iron that results could be important in explaining the degenerative changes that occur in the disease.

Specific reduction of calcium-binding protein (28-kilodalton calbindin-D) gene expression in aging and neurodegenerative diseases. Iacopino AM; Christakos S. *Proceedings of the National Academy of Sciences of the United States of America*, 1990 Jun, 87(11):4078–82.

> In Alzheimer's disease, and in aging in general, decreased levels of calcium-binding protein have been observed in humans, and in rats. Disturbances in calcium balance within nerves may be responsible for some of the degeneration seen in these conditions.

The hypothesis of zinc deficiency in the pathogenesis of neurofibrillary tangles. Constantinidis J. *Medical Hypotheses*, 1991 Aug, 35(4):319–23.

> Functional zinc decreases leading to abnormal metals reaching the brain may be responsible for a number of conditions, including Alzheimer's disease. A nontoxic zinc compound crossing the blood-brain barrier may be useful in treating Alzheimer's, which is associated with decreased levels of zinc and increased brain levels of aluminum and iron.

Thiamine and Alzheimer's disease. A pilot study. Blass JP; Gleason
P; Brush D; DiPonte P; Thaler H. *Archives of Neurology*, 1988
Aug, 45(8):833–5.

> In a double-blind, placebo-controlled study, Alzheimer's
> patients showing no signs of thiamine deficiency, but
> treated with thiamine over three months, showed
> cognitive improvements.

Vitamin B_{12} levels in serum and cerebrospinal fluid of people with
Alzheimer's disease. Ikeda T; Furukawa Y; Mashimoto S;
Takahaski K; Yamada M. *Acta Psychiatrica Scandinavica*, 1990
Oct, 82(4):327–9.

> Low levels of vitamin B_{12} in the cerebrospinal fluid of
> Alzheimer's patients are characteristic of the disease.

Vitamin B_{12}-induced reduction of platelet monoamine oxidase
activity in patients with dementia and pernicious anaemia.
Regland B; Gottfries CG; Oreland L. *European Archives of
Psychiatry and Clinical Neuroscience*, 1991, 240(4–5):288–91

> There is a significant connection between vitamin B_{12}
> deficiency and Alzheimer's disease. When Alzheimer's
> patients were treated with B_{12}, their increased platelet
> monoamine oxidase activity (a characteristic of the
> disease), was significantly reduced.

Vitamin E and Alzheimer's disease in subjects with Down's syndrome.
Jackson CV; Holland AJ; Williams CA; Dickerson JW. *Journal of
Mental Deficiency Research*, 1988 Dec, 32 (Pt 6):479–84.

> People with Down's syndrome are at high risk of
> developing Alzheimer's disease; they seem, because of
> their genetic make-up, to be more susceptible to
> oxidative damage. Blood levels of vitamin E in 12 Down's
> syndrome subjects with Alzheimer's disease were lower
> than those in 12 Down's subjects without the disease,
> suggesting an interaction between risk of Alzheimer's and
> the protective action of vitamin E against oxidative
> damage.

ANOREXIA

Evidence of zinc deficiency in anorexia nervosa and bulimia nervosa. Schauss AG; Bryce-Smith D. *Nutrients and brain function*; editor, WB Essman. Basel: Karger, c 1987. p. 151–162.

> A review is presented on the use of zinc in treating anorexia nervosa, and on the zinc taste-test for assessing zinc deficiency, which is frequent in anorexics.

Nutrition in the elderly [clinical conference]. Morley JE; Mooradian AD; Silver AJ; Heber D; Alfin-Slater RB. *Annals of Internal Medicine*, 1988 Dec 1, 109(11):890–904.

> Unrecognized depression is a common, and treatable, cause of loss of appetite in the elderly. Lack of vitamin D can be a problem, due to decreased exposure to sunlight, and lack of ability to form this vitamin. Zinc and selenium levels may be low, which can lead to deteriorating vision and increased cancer risk, respectively.

Zinc absorption in anorexia nervosa. Dinsmore, WW; Alderdice, JT; McMaster, D; Adams, CEA; Love, AH. *Lancet*. Boston, Mass.: Little, Brown and Company. May 4, 1985. v.1 (8):1041–1042.

> Anorexics have a lower intestinal uptake of zinc than do normal subjects.

ANXIETY

Effect of a herbal psychotropic preparation, BR-16A (Mentat), on performance of mice on elevated plus-maze. Verma A; Kulkarni SK. *Indian Journal of Experimental Biology*, 1991 Dec, 29(12):1120–3.

> In experiments with mice, the herbal preparation BR-16A (Mentat) was shown to reduce anxiety.

Magnesium, schizophrenia and manic-depressive disease. Kirov GK; Tsachev KN. *Neuropsychobiology*, 1990, 23(2):79–81.

> Magnesium levels in the blood of schizophrenic and

depressed patients were shown to be lower than normal. The levels increased for those schizophrenics achieving clinical remission. It is hypothesized that the high stress level in severely ill psychiatric patients can sometimes lead to magnesium deficiency, which in turn could exacerbate symptoms such as anxiety, fear, hallucinations, weakness, and physical complaints.

Pre-operative anxiety and serum potassium. McCleane GJ; Watters CH. *Anaesthesia*, 1990 Jul, 45(7):583–5.

Two hundred pre-operative patients were assessed for anxiety, and the most anxious ones showed lowered blood potassium levels.

Role of an indigenous drug geriforte on blood levels of biogenic amines and its significance in the treatment of anxiety neurosis. Upadhyaya L; Tiwari AK; Agrawal A; Dubey GP. *Activitas Nervosa Superior*, 1990 Mar, 32(1):1–5.

The herbal preparation Geriforte was found effective in reducing anxiety and stress in neurotic anxiety patients.

The impact of selenium supplementation on mood. Benton D; Cook R. *Biological Psychiatry*, 1991 Jun 1, 29(11):1092–8.

To look into the possibility that a subclinical deficiency of selenium exists in a sample of the British population, 50 subjects were given either a selenium supplement or a placebo, in a double-blind study over five weeks. The selenium was shown to elevate mood and, in particular, to decrease anxiety, and these effects were more pronounced in those subjects who had lower levels of selenium in their diets to begin with. The results are discussed in terms of the low level of selenium in the food chain in some parts of the world.

Vitamin B_{12} and folic acid serum levels in obsessive compulsive disorder. Hermesh H; Weizman A; Shahar A; Munitz H. *Acta Psychiatrica Scandinavica*, 1988 Jul, 78(1):8–10.

Vitamin B_{12} deficiency was shown to be associated with

a subgroup of patients with obsessive compulsive disorder.

Vitamin C status in chronic schizophrenia. Suboticanec K; Folnegovic-Smalc V; Korbar M; Mestrovic B; Buzina R. *Biological Psychiatry*, 1990 Dec 1, 28(11):959–66.

Schizophrenic patients on the same hospital diet as control group patients showed lower levels of vitamin C in their blood, and even when they were supplemented to normalize their blood levels of the vitamin, levels excreted in their urine remained lower than those of the control group. The results support the view that schizophrenic patients need more vitamin C than the suggested requirement for healthy people.

Effect of a special kava extract in patients with anxiety-, tension-, and excitation states of non-psychotic genesis. Double blind study with placebos over 4 weeks. (in German) Kinzler E; Kromer J; Lehmann E. *Arzneimittel-Forschung*, 1991 Jun, 41(6):584–8.

In a double-blind study, patients with anxiety syndrome not caused by psychotic disorders were treated with either kava extract or a placebo. A significant, and progressive, anxiety-reducing effect was seen for the kava over a period of four weeks. No side effects were noted.

Psychosomatic dysfunctions in the female climacteric. Clinical effectiveness and tolerance of Kava Extract WS 1490. (in German) Warnecke G. *Fortschritte der Medizin*, 1991 Feb 10, 109(4):119–22.

In a double-blind study, kava extract worked better than a placebo in relieving menopausal symptoms, and was well-tolerated.

AUTISM

Biotin-responsive infantile encephalopathy: EEG-polygraphic study of a case. Colamaria V; Burlina AB; Gaburro D; Pajno-Ferrara F; Saudubray JM; Merino RG; Dalla Bernardina B. *Epilepsia*, 1989 Sep–Oct, 30(5):573–8.

An infant suffering from autistic-like behavior, progressive lethargy, muscle spasms, generalized seizures, and other symptoms was treated with biotin twice daily and showed dramatic improvement of all symptoms.

Controversies in the treatment of autistic children: vitamin and drug therapy. Rimland B. *Journal of Child Neurology*, 1988, 3 Suppl:S68–72.

A survey of approximately 4000 questionnaires completed by parents of autistic children provided ratings of various treatments. Among the biomedical treatments, the highest-ranking one was the use of high-dosage vitamin B_6 and magnesium, with 8.5 parents reporting behavioral improvement to every one reporting behavioral worsening. The most-used drug on the list, thioridazine hydrochloride (Mellaril), came in fourth, with a helped-worsened ratio of 1.4:1.

The effects of combined pyridoxine plus magnesium administration on the conditioned evoked potentials in children with autistic behavior. Martineau J; Barthelemy C; Roux S; Lelord G. *Curr. Top. Nutr. Dis.*, New York, NY: Alan R. Liss. 1988. v.19:357–362.

Vitamin B_6 plus magnesium was shown to be effective in the treatment of autistic children.

Nutritional treatments currently under investigation in autism. Coleman M. *Clin. Nutr.*, St. Louis, MO: CV Mosby Co. Sept/ Oct 1989. v.8(5):210–212.

Autism has multiple causes, and many types of autism can be treated by nutritional approaches, e.g., the folic acid therapy of the fragile X syndrome, the low-phenylalanine diet of phenylketonuria, the restricted purine diet of purine autism, the high-calcium diet of autism with hypocalcinuria, and the ketogenic diet of autism with lactic acidosis. Such targeted therapies appear to be the future approach to autism.

Vitamin B$_6$ versus fenfluramine: A case-study in medical bias. Rimland B. *J. Nutr. Med.* Abingdon, UK: Carfax Pub. Co. 1991. v.2(3):321–322.

> Vitamin B$_6$ and magnesium—as opposed to the drug fenfluramine—constitute the first-choice treatment in the treatment of autistic children and adults.

BIPOLAR DISORDER

Abnormal intracellular calcium ion concentration in platelets and lymphocytes of bipolar patients. Dubovsky SL; Murphy J; Thomas M; Rademacher J. *American Journal of Psychiatry*, 1992 Jan, 149(1):118–20.

> There seems to be a disturbance in calcium regulation in the systems of patients with bipolar disorder.

Calcium function in affective disorders and healthy controls. Bowden CL; Huang LG; Javors MA; Johnson JM; Seleshi E; McIntyre K; Contreras S; Maas JW. *Biological Psychiatry*, 1988 Feb 15, 23(4):367–76.

> Calcium activity was shown to be abnormal in bipolar depressed and manic patients, and in unipolar patients. Also, unipolar and bipolar patients showed different types of disturbances in calcium metabolism.

Elevated platelet intracellular calcium concentration in bipolar depression. Dubovsky SL; Lee C; Christiano J; Murphy J. *Biological Psychiatry*, 1991 Mar 1, 29(5):441–50.

> It is suggested that untreated bipolar depressed patients had changes in calcium regulation within their cells that were not characteristic of untreated unipolar depressed patients.

Folate concentration in Chinese psychiatric outpatients on long-term lithium treatment. Lee S; Chow CC; Shek CC; Wing YK; Chen CN. *Journal of Affective Disorders*, 1992 Apr, 24(4):265–70.

> While folate deficiency is uncommon among Chinese

psychiatric patients, it was shown that patients with a good response to lithium treatment over one year had a higher folate level in their blood than those showing an unsatisfactory response. This supports recent evidence that folate at high concentrations enhances the benefits of lithium.

Folic acid enhances lithium prophylaxis. Coppen A; Chaudhry S; Swade C. *Journal of Affective Disorders*, 1986 Jan–Feb, 10(1):9–13.

In a double-blind study of patients on lithium therapy, those receiving a folic acid supplement showed a significant reduction of their symptoms compared to a group receiving a placebo.

Further studies of vanadium in depressive psychosis. Naylor GJ; Corrigan FM; Smith AH; Connelly P; Ward NI. *British Journal of Psychiatry*, 1987 May, 150:656–61.

Changes in tissue vanadium concentration may explain the changes in sodium transport that occur in depressive psychosis.

Incorporation of inositol into the phosphoinositides of lymphoblastoid cell lines established from bipolar manic-depressive patients. Banks RE; Aiton JF; Cramb G; Naylor GJ. *Journal of Affective Disorders*, 1990 May, 19(1):1–8.

Patients with manic-depressive disorder showed lower uptake of inositol when compared with a control group.

Lithium mechanisms in bipolar illness and altered intracellular calcium functions. Meltzer HL. *Biological Psychiatry*, 1986 May, 21(5–6):492–510.

Calcium acts between cells in a variety of ways by activating a wide range of enzymes. Since lithium seems to alter many calcium-dependent processes, it may be that bipolar illness is a result of disturbances in calcium-regulated functions.

Long-term lithium treatment. Some clinical, psychological and biological aspects. Smigan L. *Acta Psychiatrica Scandinavica*, 1985 Feb, 71(2):160–70.

> Patients with affective disorders who responded favorably to lithium treatment showed a rise in calcium levels in their blood during the first four months of treatment. Those who did not respond to lithium showed unaltered calcium levels.

Red cell folate concentrations in psychiatric patients. Carney MW: Chary TK; Laundy M; Bottiglieri T; Chanarin I; Reynolds EH; Toone B. *Journal of Affective Disorders*, 1990 Jul, 19(3):207–13.

> Depressed patients were found to have low folate levels.

The calcium second messenger system in bipolar disorders: data supporting new research directions. Dubovsky SL; Murphy J; Christiano J; Lee C. *Journal of Neuropsychiatry and Clinical Neurosciences*, 1992 Winter, 4(1):3–14.

> Irregularities in calcium's signal-sending actions within cells may explain bipolar disorders. Lithium and other mood-stabilizing treatments seem to work by regulating calcium ion hyperactivity.

The use of sodium and potassium to reduce toxicity and toxic side effects from lithium. Cater RE. *Medical Hypotheses*, 1986 Aug, 20(4):359–83.

> In rats, toxic side effects of lithium were prevented by feeding sodium and potassium. While sodium alone has been used to reduce side effects in humans, it can reduce lithium's benefits. Evidence suggests that using both sodium and potassium together would be better because the lithium dose could be slightly raised without adverse effect.

Trace elements and the electroencephalogram during long-term lithium treatment. Harvey NS: Jarratt J; Ward NI. *British Journal of Psychiatry*, 1992 May, 160:654–8.

Raised bromine levels have been found in patients during lithium treatment, and it is suggested that bromine may aid the therapeutic effect of lithium.

Vanadium and other trace elements in patients taking lithium. Campbell CA; Peet M; Ward NI. *Biological Psychiatry*, 1988 Nov, 24(7):775–81.

Compared to controls, patients on lithium had lower levels of vanadium and cobalt in their blood, and higher levels of aluminum.

Vitamin B_{12} and folate status in acute geropsychiatric inpatients: affective and cognitive characteristics of a vitamin nondeficient population. Bell IR; Edman JS; Marby DW; Satlin A; Dreier T; Liptzin B; Cole JO. *Biological Psychiatry*, 1990 Jan 15, 27(2):125–37.

A study was done of geriatric patients admitted to a psychiatric hospital. Although they were not generally vitamin-deficient, those with below-median values of vitamin B_{12} and folate had more severe psychiatric problems than those with higher levels of one or both vitamins. It is suggested that biochemically interrelated vitamins such as B_{12} and folate may exert both a separate and combined influence on mental state, and that poorer vitamin status may contribute to some psychiatric disorders in the elderly.

Vitamin B_6 in clinical neurology. Bernstein AL. *Annals of the New York Academy of Sciences*, 1990, 585:250–60.

Vitamin B_6 supplementation may be useful in treating a number of conditions. For instance, headache, chronic pain, and depression, all associated with serotonin deficiency, have, in some studies, been shown to have been helped by B_6, which raises serotonin levels. In addition, B_6 may reverse the effects of toxic substances associated with hyperactivity and aggressive behavior.

BULIMIA

Plasma and cerebrospinal fluid measures of arginine vasopressin secretion in patients with bulimia nervosa and in healthy subjects. Demitrack MA; Kalogeras KT; Altemus M; Pigott TA; Listwak SJ; Gold PW. *Journal of Clinical Endocrinology and Metabolism*, 1992 Jun, 74(6):1277–83.

> Normal-weight female bulimic patients who had abstained from binge eating and purging for at least a month were studied. It was shown that they had irregularities in the hormonal process that regulates fluid volume in the body, a fact that may be relevant to their behavior.

The effect of bulimia upon diet, body fat, bone density, and blood components. Howat PM; Varner LM; Hegsted M; Brewer MM; Mills GQ. *Journal of the American Dietetic Association*, 1989 Jul, 89(7):929–34.

> Bulimic subjects were compared with controls, and it was found that the bulimics' folacin intake was significantly lower than that of the controls. Also, the bulimics consumed lower quantities of vitamin/mineral supplements, and their bone minieral densities and hemoglobin levels were lower.

Zinc deficiency and eating disorders. Humphries L; Vivian B; Stuart M; McClain CJ. *Journal of Clinical Psychiatry*, 1989 Dec, 50(12):456–9.

> Zinc status was evaluated in bulimic and anorexic patients, many of whom were found to be deficient in the mineral. This is due to a variety of reasons—lower dietary intake of zinc, impaired absorption, vomiting, diarrhea, and binging on low-zinc foods. Since zinc deficiency results in decreased food intake, the acquired zinc deficiency of bulimics and anorexics could exacerbate their altered eating behavior.

Zinc status before and after zinc supplementation of eating disorder patients. McClain CJ; Stuart MA; Vivian B; McClain M; Talwalker R; Snelling L; Humphries L. *Journal of the American College of Nutrition*, 1992 Dec, 11(6):694–700.

> Since reduced food intake results from zinc deficiency, the acquired zinc deficiency of eating disorder patients may act as a sustaining factor for their abnormal eating behavior. Hospitalized bulimics and anorexics were shown to be deficient in the mineral, and to benefit from supplementation.

CANDIDA

Allium sativum (garlic) inhibits lipid synthesis by Candida albicans. Adetumbi M; Javor GT; Lau BH. *Antimicrobial Agents and Chemotherapy*, 1986 Sep, 30(3):499–501.

> Garlic extract was shown to inhibit the proliferation of the Candida albicans fungus.

Carrot phytoalexin alters the membrane permeability of Candida albicans and multilamellar liposomes. Amin M; Kurosaki F; Nishi A. *Journal of General Microbiology*, 1988 Jan, 134 (Pt 1):241–6.

> Carrots have an ingredient that inhibits the candida organism by damaging its cell membranes.

Effect of calcium ion uptake on Candida albicans morphology. Holmes AR; Cannon RD; Shepherd MG. *Fems Microbiology Letters*, 1991 Jan 15, 61(2–3):187–93.

> Calcium was shown to inhibit the growth of Candida albicans yeast cells.

Inhibition of Candida adhesion to buccal epithelial cells by an aqueous extract of Allium sativum (garlic). Ghannoum MA. *Journal of Applied Bacteriology*, 1990 Feb, 68(2):163–9.

> Garlic extract inhibits the adhesion of candida cells to human cells taken from the inside of the cheek.

Respiratory burst and candidacidal activity of peritoneal macrophages are impaired in copper-deficient rats. Babu U; Failla ML. *Journal of Nutrition*, 1990 Dec, 120(12):1692–9.

> In rats, a copper-deficient diet resulted in reduced resistance to candida cells. Rats fed a diet with adequate copper, by contrast, had better systemic defenses against candida.

Studies on the anticandidal mode af action of Allium sativum (garlic). Ghannoum MA. *Journal of General Microbiology*, 1988 Nov, 134 (Pt 11):2917–24.

> Garlic extract slows the growth of Candida albicans by affecting the outer surface of the cells and reducing their oxygen consumption, among other means.

DEMENTIA

Calcium and phosphorus levels in serum and CSF in dementia. Subhash MN; Padmashree TS; Srinivas KN; Subbakrishna DK; Shankar SK. *Neurobiology of Aging*, 1991 Jul–Aug, 12(4):267–9.

> There is a significant decrease in levels of calcium and phosphorus in the cerebrospinal fluid of patients with Alzheimer's-type dementia and in dementia caused by blood-vessel disease or stroke. The drops in the levels of these minerals in the patient groups go beyond those associated with normal aging.

Cephaloconiosis: a free radical perspective on the proposed particulate-induced etiopathogenesis of Alzheimer's dementia and related disorders. Evans PH; Klinowski J; Yano E. *Medical Hypotheses*, 1991 Mar, 34(3):209–19.

> It is suggested that Alzheimer's dementia and related disorders are caused by fiber-like deposits of inorganic substances in the brain. Antioxidants—either micronutrients or pharmacological agents—may be therapeutic.

Double-blind, placebo controlled study of acetyl-l-carnitine in patients with Alzheimer's dementia. Rai G; Wright G; Scott L; Beston B; Rest J; Exton-Smith AN. *Current Medical Research and Opinion*, 1990, 11(10):638–47.

> Patients with Alzheimer's-type dementia were treated with acetyl-l-carnitine and compared with a control group. The treated group showed less deterioration than did the group receiving placebos, particularly in the area of short-term memory.

Low serum cobalamin levels in primary degenerative dementia. Do some patients harbor atypical cobalamin deficiency states? Karnaze DS; Carmel R. *Archives of Internal Medicine*, 1987 Mar, 147(3):429–31.

> Low levels of vitamin B_{12} in the blood are frequent in cases of primary degenerative dementia.

Treatment of Alzheimer-type dementia with intravenous mecobalamin. Ikeda T; Yamamoto K; Takahashi K; Kaku Y; Uchiyama M; Sugiyama K; Yamada M. *Clinical Therapeutics*, 1992 May–Jun, 14(3):426–37.

> Intravenous mecobalamin was seen to be a safe and effective treatment for patients with Alzheimer's-type dementia; it improved intellectual functions, such as memory, as well as emotional functions and communication abilities.

DEPRESSION

Acute antidepressant effect of lithium is associated with fluctuation of calcium and magnesium in plasma. A double-blind study on the antidepressant effect of lithium and clomipramine. Linder J; Fyro B; Pettersson U; Werner S. *Acta Psychiatrica Scandinavica*, 1989 Jul, 80(1):27–36.

> Lithium treatment of patients with major depressive disorder was associated with fluctuations in blood calcium and magnesium levels. These fluctuations were

not seen in treatment with the drug clomipramine.

Erythrocyte electrolytes in psychiatric illness. Esche I; Joffe RT; Blank DW. *Acta Psychiatrica Scandinavica*, 1988 Dec, 78(6):695–7.

Fluctuations in sodium and potassium were found within the red blood cells of patients with psychiatric disorders experiencing changes in mood state. These fluctuations were not found in a healthy control group.

Levels of copper and zinc in depression. Narang RL; Gupta KR: Narang AP; Singh R. *Indian Journal of Physiology and Pharmacology*, 1991 Oct, 35(4):272–4.

Copper levels in depressed patients were significantly higher than those in controls, as well as higher than those in the same patients after they had recovered from depression. Zinc levels in depressed patients were not significantly lower than those of controls, but they were significantly lower than those of the same patients once they had recovered.

Myths about vitamin B_{12} deficiency. Fine EJ; Soria ED. *Southern Medical Journal*, 1991 Dec, 84(12):1475–81.

Deficiency of vitamin B_{12} can cause nerve problems, depression, and dementia. Vitamin B_{12} replacement should be given to patients with borderline levels of the vitamin, since the advantages of doing so outweigh any disadvantages of therapy.

Nutritional aspects of psychiatric disorders. Gray GE; Gray LK. *J Am Diet Assoc.* Chicago, Ill.: The Association. Oct 1989. v.89(10):1492–8.

Dietitians have a role as part of a multidisciplinary team in the treatment of psychiatric patients. Psychiatric illnesses may adversely affect food intake and nutritional status. Also, the drugs used to treat the disorders, including antipsychotics, antidepressants, monoamine oxidase inhibitors, and lithium, can affect appetite and gastrointestinal function, and can interact with foods.

Study of the efficacy and tolerability of L-acetylcarnitine therapy in the senile brain. Bonavita E. *International Journal of Clinical Pharmacology, Therapy, and Toxicology*, 1986 Sep, 24(9):511–6.

> A double-blind, placebo-controlled study showed that treatment with L-acetylcarnitine can improve the mental abilities of senile patients.

The biology of folate in depression: implications for nutritional hypotheses of the psychoses. Abou-Saleh MT; Coppen A. *Journal of Psychiatric Research*, 1986, 20(2):91–101.

> Folate deficiency is common in psychiatric disorders, particularly depression. This deficiency—with or without deficiencies of other nutritional factors—may predispose people to psychiatric disturbances, or may worsen existing conditions.

Zinc in depressive disorder. McLoughlin IJ; Hodge JS. *Acta Psychiatrica Scandinavica*, 1990 Dec, 82(6):451–3.

> Levels of zinc in the blood of patients admitted to a hospital for depression were lower than those in a control group. Upon release from the hospital after treatment, the patients' zinc levels had gone up significantly.

EATING DISORDERS

Anorexia nervosa responding to zinc supplementation: a case report. Yamaguchi H; Arita Y; Hara Y; Kimura T; Nawata H. *Gastroenterologia Japonica*, 1992 Aug, 27(4):554–8.

> Zinc supplementation may be a therapeutic option in anorexia. In an anorexic patient with a low zinc level, supplementary zinc was given. The patient's digestive symptoms disappeared, and she regained normal weight.

Oral zinc supplementation in anorexia nervosa. Safai-Kutti S. *Acta Psychiatrica Scandinavica*. Supplementum, 1990, 361:14–7.

> There is evidence to suggest that zinc deficiency is a causative factor in anorexia nervosa. Anorexic patients

receiving zinc supplementation showed weight gain. The design of a placebo-controlled study of zinc supplementation in anorexia is described.

Treatment of childhood anorexia with spleen deficiency by Qiang Zhuang Ling. Zou ZW; Li XM. *Journal of Traditional Chinese Medicine*, 1989 Jun, 9(2):100–2.

The traditional Chinese herbal prescription Qiang Zhuang Ling was used to treat a group of patients suffering from childhood anorexia with spleen deficiency. The therapeutic effect of the herbs was significantly greater than that seen in another group of patients treated with a zinc sulphate solution.

Zinc deficiency and childhood-onset anorexia nervosa. Lask B; Fosson A; Rolfe U; Thomas S. *Journal of Clinical Psychiatry*, 1993 Feb, 54(2):63–6.

Zinc deficiency was found to be common in childhood-onset anorexia nervosa.

Zinc status in anorexia nervosa. Varela P; Marcos A; Navarro MP. *Annals of Nutrition and Metabolism*, 1992, 36(4):197–202.

The body's zinc-dependent functions may be impaired in anorexia nervosa as a consequence of zinc unavailability.

HYPERKINESIS

Developmental effects of vitamin B_6 restriction on the locomotor behavior of rats. Guilarte TR; Miceli RC; Moran TH. *Brain Research Bulletin*, 1991 Jun, 26(6):857–61.

Newborn rats on a vitamin-B_6-restricted diet were less active than those in a control group. However, when the vitamin-B_6-deprived rats got older, they became hyperactive. Long-term B_6 deprivation seems to result in damage to the nerve systems associated with locomotor behavior.

Neonatal hyperexcitability in relation to plasma ionized calcium, magnesium, phosphate and glucose. Nelson N; Finnstrom O; Larsson L. *Acta Paediatrica Scandinavica*, 1987 Jul, 76(4):579–84.

> Newborn, full-term babies who seemed hyperactive at birth were shown to have low magnesium levels. The levels normalized spontaneously at five days of age.

Vitamin B_{12} improves cognitive disturbance in rodents fed a choline-deficient diet. Sasaki H; Matsuzaki Y; Meguro K; Ikarashi Y; Maruyama Y; Yamaguchi S; Sekizawa K. *Pharmacology, Biochemistry and Behavior*, 1992 Oct, 43(2):635–9.

> Rats on a choline-deficient diet were less able to learn than rats on a choline-enriched diet. However, when the choline-deficient diet was supplemented with vitamin B_{12}, there were no differences in learning ability between the groups.

Subtle abnormalities of gait detected early in vitamin B_6 deficiency in aged and weanling rats with hind leg gait analysis. Schaeffer MC; Cochary EF; Sadowski JA. *Journal of the American College of Nutrition*, 1990 Apr, 9(2):120–7.

> Motor abnormalities have been observed in every species made vitamin-B_6-deficient. In rats, a deficiency of the vitamin is reflected in an abnormal gait at 2–3 weeks of age.

INSOMNIA

Double blind study of a valerian preparation. Lindahl O; Lindwall L. *Pharmacology, Biochemistry and Behavior*, 1989 Apr, 32(4):1065–6.

> A valerian root preparation was compared with a placebo in a double-blind test of its sedative effects. It showed significant effectiveness in improving sleep, and no side effects were observed.

Neuropsychopharmacologic properties of a Schumanniophyton problematicum root extract. Amadi E; Offiah NV; Akah PA. *Journal of Ethnopharmacology*, 1991 May–Jun, 33(1–2):73–7.

An extract of Schumanniophyton problematicum, a plant popular among Nigerian native healers for the treatment of psychosis, was given to mice. The extract, which appears to depress the central and autonomic nervous systems, can inhibit hyperactivity caused by amphetamines, induce passivity, and prolong sleeping time induced by the tranquilizer pentobarbital.

Neurotropic action of the hydroalcoholic extract of Melissa officinalis in the mouse. Soulimani R; Fleurentin J; Mortier F; Misslin R; Derrieu G; Pelt JM. *Planta Medica*, 1991 Apr, 57(2):105–9.

An extract of Melissa officinalis was tested in mice and shown to have sedative properties at low doses, and pain-relieving and sleep-inducing properties at higher doses.

Panax ginseng extract modulates sleep in unrestrained rats. Rhee YH; Lee SP; Honda K; Inoue S. *Psychopharmacology*, 1990, 101(4):486–8.

Panax ginseng extract was found to enhance the amount of slow-wave sleep in rats.

Parasomnias (non-epileptic nocturnal episodic manifestations) in patients with magnesium deficiency. Popoviciu L; Delast-Popoviciu D; Delast-Popoviciu R; Bagathai I; Bicher G; Buksa C; Covaciu S; Szalay E. *Romainian Journal of Neurology and Psychiatry*, 1990 Jan–Mar, 28(1):19–24.

Severe sleep disorders, such as night terrors, may be linked to brain damage caused by magnesium deficiency.

Pharmacological investigations on Achyrocline satureioides (LAM.) DC., Compositae. Simoes CM; Schenkel EP; Bauer L; Langeloh A. *Journal of Ethnopharmacology*, 1988 Apr, 22(3):281–93.

Among the therapeutic properties of Achyrocline satureioides (Lam.) DC. is its sleep-enhancing effect, which was shown in mice.

Potassium affects actigraph-identified sleep. Drennan MD; Kripke DF; Klemfuss HA; Moore JD. *Sleep*, 1991 Aug, 14(4):357–60.

A double-blind, placebo-controlled study with normal young males on a low-potassium diet showed that potassium supplements may increase sleep efficiency, lessening the frequency of wakefulness immediately after the onset of sleep.

Preliminary psychopharmacological evaluation of Ocimum sanctum leaf extract. Sakina MR; Dandiya PC; Hamdard ME; Hameed A. *Journal of Ethnopharmacology*, 1990 Feb, 28(2):143–50.

An extract of the leaves of Ocimum sanctum was shown in mice to have a sedative effect.

Psychotropic effects of Japanese valerian root extract. Sakamoto T; Mitani Y; Nakajima K. *Chemical and Pharmaceutical Bulletin*, 1992 Mar, 40(3):758–61.

Valerian extract, which acts on the central nervous system, was shown to prolong drug-induced sleep in mice. The extract may also be an antidepressant.

Treatment of persistent sleep-wake schedule disorders in adolescents with methylcobalamin (vitamin B_{12}). Ohta T; Ando K; Iwata T; Ozaki N; Kayukawa Y; Terashima M; Okada T; Kasahara Y. *Sleep*, 1991 Oct, 14(5):414–8.

Two adolescents suffering from persistent sleep-wake rhythm disorders were helped by treatment with vitamin B_{12}, although neither had shown evidence of B_{12} deficiency, or of hypothyroidism, which can cause deficiency.

Vitamin B_{12} treatment for sleep-wake rhythm disorders. Okawa M; Mishima K; Nanami T; Shimizu T; Ijima S; Hishikawa Y; Takahashi K. *Sleep*, 1990 Feb, 13(1):15–23.

Patients with sleep-wake schedule disorders were helped

by daily administration of vitamin B_{12}. (Blood levels of the vitamin were within the normal range before treatment.)

Neuro-depressive properties of essential oil of lavender. (in French) Delaveau P; Guillemain J; Narcisse G; Rousseau A. *Comptes Rendus des Seances de la Societe de Biologie et de Sesfiliales*, 1989, 183(4):342–8.

Essential oil of lavender given to mice relieves anxiety and prolongs drug-induced sleeping time, although only for the first five days it is administered.

Neurodepressive effects of the essential oil of Lavandula angustifolia Mill. (In French) Guillemain J; Rousseau A; Delaveau P. *Annales Pharmaceutiques Francaises*, 1989, 47(6):337–43.

Oil of lavender given to mice produced a sedative effect.

Quality of Schisandra incarnata Stapf. (in Chinese) Song W. *Chung-Kuo Chung Yao Tsa Chih China Journal of Chinese Materiamedica*, 1991 Apr, 16(4):204–6, 253.

The medicinal plant Schisandra incarnata has sleep-enhancing properties.

LEARNING DISORDERS AND DYSLEXIA

Learning and memory disabilities in young adult rats from mildly zinc deficient dams. Halas ES; Hunt CD; Eberhardt MJ. *Physiology and Behavior*, 1986, 37(3):451–8.

Rats whose mothers had had a mildly zinc-deficient diet during pregnancy and lactation were shown to have a learning deficit in that their short-term memory was impaired.

The effects of acetyl-l-carnitine on experimental models of learning and memory deficits in the old rat. Valerio C; Clementi G; Spadaro F; D'Agata V; Raffaele R; Grassi M; Lauria N; Drago F. *Functional Neurology*, 1989 Oct–Dec, 4(4):387–90.

Aged rats, which generally have impaired learning and memory capacity, were treated with acetyl-l-carnitine. They showed significant improvement in these areas.

ORGANIC MENTAL DISORDERS

Acetyl-L-carnitine in the treatment of midly demented elderly patients. Passeri M; Cucinotta D; Bonati PA; Iannuccelli M; Parnetti L; Senin U. *International Journal of Clinical Pharmacology Research*, 1990, 10(1–2):75–9.

> In a double-blind study, acetyl-L-carnitine, which acts to alleviate defects in nerve signals, was shown to help mildly demented elderly patients in the areas of behavior, memory, attention, and verbal fluency.

Acute organic psychosis caused by thyrotoxicosis and vitamin B_{12} deficiency: case report. Lassen E; Ewald H. *Journal of Clinical Psychiatry*, 1985 Mar, 46(3):106–7

> A patient developed an acute psychosis due to a deficiency of thyroid hormone and vitamin B_{12}. Replacement of thyroid hormone and B_{12} corrected the condition.

Alterations in calcium content and biochemical processes in cultured skin fibroblasts from aged and Alzheimer donors. Peterson C; Goldman JE. *Proceedings of the National Academy of Sciences of the United States of America*, 1986 Apr, 83(8):2758–62.

> Calcium balance and certain functions within cells are altered in both aging and Alzheimer's disease, but they are altered more in Alzheimer's than in normal aging.

Biological effects of aging on bone and the central nervous system. Fujita T. *Experimental Gerontology*, 1990, 25(3–4):317–21.

> The most common diseases of the elderly are osteoporosis and senile dementia. These conditions may be related in that abnormalities of calcium metabolism affect both the skeletal and nervous systems.

Cerebral atrophy and hypoperfusion improve during treatment of Wernicke-Korsakoff syndrome. Meyer JS; Tanahashi N; Ishikawa Y; Hata T; Velez M; Fann WE; Kandula P; Mortel KF; Rogers RL. *Journal of Cerebral Blood Flow and Metabolism*, 1985 Sep, 5(3):376–85.

> Early recognition and treatment of Wernicke-Korsakoff syndrome improves patients' cognitive and neurological impairments rapidly. Treatment includes alcohol withdrawal, nutritious diet, and thiamine supplements.

Clinical signs in the Wernicke-Korsakoff complex: a retrospective analysis of 131 cases diagnosed at necropsy. Harper CG: Giles M; Finlay-Jones R. *Journal of Neurology, Neurosurgery and Psychiatry*, 1986 Apr, 49(4):341–5.

> Alcoholics are at risk of Wernicke-Korsakoff syndrome, which often goes undiagnosed. Repeated episodes of vitamin B_1 deficiency may be the cause of the syndrome, and alcoholics should be monitored for this.

Cytosolic free calcium and cell spreading decrease in fibroblasts from aged and Alzheimer donors. Peterson C; Ratan RR; Shelanski ML; Goldman JE. *Proceedings of the National Academy of Sciences of the United States of America*, 1986 Oct, 83(20):7999–8001.

> At the cellular level, Alzheimer's disease is not just a cerebral disease, but a systemic one: Alterations in calcium regulation are found throughout the body. These alterations are found in normal elderly people as well, but not to the same extent as in Alzheimer's patients. Some of the cellular changes in Alzheimer's patients can be partially reversed by treatment with a form of calcium.

Disappearance of high-incidence amyotrophic lateral sclerosis and parkinsonism-dementia on Guam. Garruto RM; Yanagihara R; Gajdusek DC. *Neurology*, 1985 Feb, 35(2):193–8.

> Nutritional deficiencies of calcium and magnesium, with resultant deposition of calcium and aluminum in

neurons, may have been factors in the high rates of amyotrophic lateral sclerosis and parkinsonism-dementia that occurred several decades ago among the Chamorros of Guam.

Efficacy and clinical relevance of cognition enhancers. Herrmann WM; Stephan K. *Alzheimer Disease and Associated Disorders*, 1991, 5 Suppl 1:S7–12.

The cognition-enhancers piracetam, acetyl-L-carnitine, and nimodipine are more effective than placebos in improving the mental functioning of patients suffering from Alzheimer's and other age-related dementias.

Neurochemical hypothesis: participation by aluminum in producing critical mass of colocalized errors in brain leads to neurological disease. Joshi JG. *Comparative Biochemistry and Physiology. C:Comparative Pharmacology*, 1991, 100(1–2):103–5.

Aluminum interferes with metabolism of glucose and of iron, as well as other functions. Metabolic errors induced by aluminum in specific areas of the brain to which the metal can be transported may lead to neurological disorders.

Neuropsychiatric aspects of trace elements. Linter CM. *British Journal of Hospital Medicine*, 1985 Dec, 34(6):361–5.

Trace elements may be causative or therapeutic factors in a wide range of illnesses. Knowledge of trace element metabolism has increased dramatically in the past decade.

Neuropsychiatric disorders caused by cobalamin deficiency in the absence of anemia or macrocytosis. Lindenbaum J; Healton EB; Savage DG; Brust JC; Garrett TJ; Podell ER; Marcell PD; Stabler SP; Allen RH. *New England Journal of Medicine*, 1988 Jun 30, 318(26):1720–8.

Neuropsychiatric disorders due to cobalamin deficiency occur commonly in the absence of anemia. Cobalamin therapy is helpful in reducing neuropsychiatric abnormalities in these cases.

Neuropsychological changes in demented patients treated with acetyl-L-carnitine. Sinforiani E; Iannuccelli M; Mauri M; Costa A; Merlo P; Bono G; Nappi G. *International Journal of Clinical Pharmacology Research*, 1990, 10(1–2):69–74.

> Patients suffering mild to moderate dementia were treated with acetyl-L-carnitine or piracetam. Significant improvement was shown in the acetyl-L-carnitine group—but not in the piracetam group—in the areas of behavior, attention, and psychomotor performance.

Pathological brain ageing: evaluation of the efficacy of a pharmacological aid. Guarnaschelli C; Fugazza G; Pistarini C. *Drugs under Experimental and Clinical Research*, 1988, 14(11):715–8.

> L-acetylcarnitine given to aged patients was shown to be effective in enhancing cognitive ability, motor activity, and self-sufficiency, and in relieving depression.

Pernicious anemia in the demented patient without anemia or macrocytosis. A case for early recognition. Gross JS; Weintraub NT; Neufeld RR; Libow LS. *Journal of the American Geriatrics Society*, 1986 Aug, 34(8):612–4.

> Pernicious anemia in elderly patients suffering from dementia can occur in the absence of anemia. Treatment with vitamin B_{12} has a therapeutic effect.

Pharmaco-electroencephalographic and clinical effects of the cholinergic substance—acetyl-L-carnitine—in patients with organic brain syndrome. Hermann WM; Dietrich B; Hiersemenzel R. *International Journal of Clinical Pharmacology Research*, 1990, 10(1–2):81–4.

> Acetyl-L-carnitine is promising as a treatment for elderly patients with impaired brain function, as shown in two double-blind, placebo-controlled studies. Side effects were not generally seen.

Pyridoxine, ascorbic acid and thiamine in Alzheimer and comparison subjects. Agbayewa MO; Bruce VM; Siemens V. *Canadian Journal of Psychiatry. Revue Canadienne de Psychiatrie*, 1992 Nov, 37(9):661–2.

> A group of patients with Alzheimer's disease showed lower functional levels of vitamin B_1 than those of a group of normal subjects.

Reduced gastrointestinal absorption of calcium in dementia. Ferrier IN; Leake A; Taylor GA; McKeith IG; Fairbairn AF; Robinson CJ; Francis RM; Edwardson JA. *Age and Ageing*, 1990 Nov, 19(6):368–75.

> Patients suffering from Alzheimer-type dementia and multi-infarct dementia showed reduced ability to absorb calcium intestinally.

Relationship of normal serum vitamin B_{12} and folate levels to cognitive test performance in subtypes of geriatric major depression. Bell IR; Edman JS; Miller J; Hebben N; Linn RT; Ray D; Kayne HL. *Journal of Geriatric Psychiatry and Neurology*, 1990 Apr–Jun, 3(2):98–105.

> Elderly patients with psychotic depression were assessed for vitamin B_{12} and folate levels. Those with higher B_{12} levels tended to do better on measures of cognitive ability. Metabolic factors, including B_{12}, may play specific roles in psychiatric disorders of the elderly.

PREMENSTRUAL SYNDROME

Assessment of magnesium status. Elin RJ. *Clinical Chemistry*, 1987 Nov, 33(11):1965–70.

> Assessing the magnesium status of an individual is difficult: Most data are taken from blood tests, yet most of the magnesium in the body is in bone and soft tissues. A better understanding of magnesium transport and metabolism is needed, as changes in magnesium status have been implicated in a number of conditions,

including heart conditions, high blood pressure, and premenstrual syndrome.

Calcium supplementation in premenstrual syndrome: a randomized crossover trial. Thys-Jacobs S; Ceccarelli S; Bierman A; Weisman H; Cohen MA; Alvir J. *Journal of General Internal Medicine,* 1989 May–Jun, 4(3):183–9.

> In a double-blind study, daily calcium supplementation was given to women suffering from premenstrual syndrome. The calcium was shown to be an effective treatment for premenstrual symptoms, including water retention and pain. It also alleviated menstrual pain.

Clinical and biochemical effects of nutritional supplementation on the premenstrual syndrome. Stewart A. *Journal of Reproductive Medicine,* 1987 Jun, 32(6):435–41.

> A study of women with premenstrual syndrome showed frequent nutritional deficiencies, particularly of vitamin B_6 and magnesium. A multivitamin and mineral supplement corrected some of the deficiencies and improved the symptoms of premenstrual tension.

Controlled trial of pyridoxine in the premenstrual syndrome. Williams MJ; Harris RI; Dean BC. *Journal of International Medical Research,* 1985, 13(3):174–9.

> Pyridoxine, compared with a placebo, was effective in alleviating premenstrual symptoms.

Effect of a nutritional supplement on premenstrual symptomatology in women with premenstrual syndrome: a double-blind longitudinal study. London RS; Bradley L; Chiamori NY. *Journal of the American College of Nutrition,* 1991 Oct, 10(5):494–9.

> Nutritional supplements proved more effective than a placebo in relieving premenstrual syndrome.

Efficacy of alpha-tocopherol in the treatment of the premenstrual syndrome. London RS; Murphy L; Kitlowski KE; Reynolds MA. *Journal of Reproductive Medicine,* 1987 Jun, 32(6):400–4.

Daily alpha-tocopherol supplements were shown to be effective in reducing premenstrual symptoms in a double-blind, placebo-controlled study.

Magnesium and the premenstrual syndrome. Sherwood RA; Rocks BF; Stewart A; Saxton RS. *Annals of Clinical Biochemistry*, 1986 Nov, 23 (Pt 6):667–70.

Women with premenstrual syndrome had significantly lower than normal levels of magnesium in their red blood cells.

Oral magnesium successfully relieves premenstrual mood changes. Facchinetti F; Borella P; Sances G; Fioroni L; Nappi RE; Genazzani AR. *Obstetrics and Gynecology*, 1991 Aug, 78(2):177–81.

Magnesium supplementation, when compared with a placebo, was effective in relieving premenstrual mood changes.

Premenstrual and menstrual symptom clusters and response to calcium treatment. Alvir JM; Thys-Jacobs S. *Psychopharmacology Bulletin*, 1991, 27(2):145–8.

Calcium supplementation was shown to alleviate three premenstrual symptoms—mood changes, water retention, and pain—and to relieve menstrual pain.

Premenstrual syndrome. Tactics for intervention. Havens C. *Postgraduate Medicine*, 1985 May 15, 77(7):32–7.

Nutritional supplements are sometimes appropriate in the treatment of premenstrual syndrome, along with dietary changes, regular exercise, and, at times, diuretics and other drugs. Vitamin B_6, and possibly vitamin E or zinc sulfate, may be used.

Pyridoxine (vitamin B_6) and the premenstrual syndrome: a randomized crossover trial. Doll H; Brown S; Thurston A; Vessey M. *Journal of the Royal College of General Practitioners*, 1989 Sep, 39(326):364–8.

In a double-blind, placebo-controlled study, vitamin B_6 supplementation was shown to be effective in alleviating emotional symptoms of premenstrual syndrome. Depression, irritability, and tiredness were reduced in women taking B_6.

Pyridoxine in the treatment of premenstrual syndrome: a retrospective survey in 630 patients. Brush MG; Bennett T; Hansen K. *British Journal of Clinical Practice*, 1988 Nov, 42(11):448–52.

Vitamin B_6 supplements seemed to be beneficial in alleviating premenstrual symptoms, according to a retrospective study. No side effects of the treatment were reported.

SCHIZOPHRENIA

Acetazolamide and thiamine: an ancillary therapy for chronic mental illness. Sacks W; Esser AH; Feitel B; Abbott K. *Psychiatry Research*, 1989 Jun, 28(3):279–88.

Treatment of chronic schizophrenic patients with the drug acetazolamide, plus thiamine, was shown to be effective on a number of assessment scales. No untoward effects were seen for this therapy.

Enhancement of recovery from psychiatric illness by methylfolate. Godfrey PS; Toone BK; Carney MW; Flynn TG; Bottiglieri T; Laundy M. Chanarin I; Reynolds EH. *Lancet*,1990 Aug 18, 336(8712):392–5.

One third of a group of psychiatric patients with either major depression or schizophrenia showed signs of folate deficiency, and took part in a double-blind, placebo-controlled study of methylfolate supplementation (in addition to standard treatment). Both depressed and schizophrenic patients showed significantly improved clinical and social recovery with the supplements, and the differences between the outcomes of the methylfolate- and placebo-receiving groups increased over time. These findings add to the evidence that disturbances of methylation in the nervous system may be a factor in some forms of mental illness.

Plasma levels and urinary vitamin C excretion in schizophrenic patients. Suboticanec K; Folnegovic-Smalc V; Turcin R; Mestrovic B; Buzina R. *Human Nutrition. Clinical Nutrition*, 1986 Nov, 40(6):421–8.

Schizophrenia may be associated with impaired ascorbic acid metabolism. Schizophrenic patients were shown to have lower vitamin C levels than those of a nonschizophrenic group of psychiatric patients that had been on the same hospital diet as the schizophrenics for at least two months. Even when the schizophrenics were given vitamin C supplements to raise their levels to those of the other group, they excreted less of the vitamin in their urine.

Pyridoxine improves drug-induced parkinsonism and psychosis in a schizophrenic patient. Sandyk R; Pardeshi R. *International Journal of Neuroscience*, 1990 Jun, 52(3–4):225–32.

Pyridoxine supplementation should be considered in psychiatric patients with drug-induced movement disorders, such as Parkinsonism and tardive dyskinesia. An underlying pyridoxine deficiency in these patients may increase the risk of these drug-induced disorders, as well as worsen psychotic behavior. The effects of pyridoxine on movement disorders, and on psychosis, seem related to its enhancing serotonin and melatonin functions.

Subacute combined degeneration of the spinal cord due to folate defiency in association with a psychotic illness. Donnelly S; Callaghan N. *Irish Medical Journal*, 1990 Jun, 83(2):73–4.

A dietary deficiency of folic acid in a psychotic patient caused spinal cord degeneration. Treatment with folic acid relieved this problem significantly, and may have contributed to an improvement in the patient's psychiatric illness.

The biology of folate in depression: implications for nutritional hypotheses of the psychoses. Abou-Saleh MT; Coppen A. *Journal of Psychiatric Research*, 1986, 20(2):91–101.

> Folate deficiency is common in psychiatric disorders, particularly in depressive illness. Alcoholic, lithium-treated, and anorexic patients are often folate-deficient. Folate deficiency—with or without deficiencies of other nutritional factors—may predispose people to psychiatric disturbances, or aggravate existing disturbances.

Unification of the findings in schizophrenia by reference to the effects of gestational zinc deficiency. Andrews RC. *Medical Hypotheses*, 1990 Feb, 31(2):141–53.

> It is hypothesized that schizophrenia is caused by the action of gestational zinc deficiency—which may or may not be caused by diet—on genetically susceptible fetuses. A nongenetic but nevertheless transmissible immune defect may play a role in this disorder.

BIOGRAPHIES AND ADDRESSES OF THE PHYSICIANS

(Where biographies of contributing physicians are not followed by addresses and/or phone numbers, this is at the request of the contributor.)

Robert C. Atkins, M.D. graduated from Cornell University Medical College and has hospital affiliations with both Columbia and Rochester universities. He is the Founder and Executive Medical Director of the Atkins Centers for Complementary Medicine, established in 1970, and President of the Foundation for the Advancement of Innovative Medicine. Among his many best-selling books is the classic *Dr. Atkins' Diet Revolution*. He specializes in treating a wide variety of disorders, including asthma, cancer, chronic fatigue, hypoglycemia and immune system disorders.

152 E. 55th St.
New York, N.Y. 10022
Tel: (212) 758-2110

Sidney M. Baker, M.D. is a practicing physician with an interest in nutritional, biochemical and environmental aspects of chronic illness in adults and children. Since leaving the full time faculty in Medical Computer Sciences at Yale Medical School in 1971, he has specialized in computer applications that help the clinician maintain accurate, detailed, structured medical records to enhance the ability of doctors to make clinical portraits of patients both as individuals and as groups.

Harold Buttram, M.D. specializes in family practice, environmental medicine, nutrition-based modalities and the treatment of allergies.

> 5724 Clymer Rd.
> Quakertown, PA 18951
> Tel: (215) 536-1890

Christopher Calapai, M.D. is an osteopathic physician board certified in family practice. He specializes in a variety of treatment modalities, including the use of intravenous vitamin therapy, chelation therapy and reconstructive nerve therapy.

> 1900 Hempstead Turnpike
> E. Meadow, N.Y. 11554
> Tel: (516) 794-0404
>   or
> 18 E. 53rd St., 3rd Fl.
> New York, N.Y. 10022
> Tel: (212)838-9100

Hyla Cass, M.D. is a holistic psychiatrist who integrates psychotherapy and nutritional medicine in her Santa Monica-based practice. In addition to being a media and corporate consultant, speaker, and seminar leader, she is an Assistant Clinical Professor of Psychiatry at UCLA School of Medicine.

> 2730 Wilshire Blvd., #301
> Santa Monica, CA 90403
> Tel: (310) 459-9866; fax: (310) 459-9466

Leander T. Ellis, M.D. is a board certified psychiatrist who has, for over 25 years, studied the effect of allergies, infections, nutrition, and other physical factors on emotional conditions such as anxiety, depression, autism, and auto-immune diseases.

Beekman Place
2746 Belmont Ave.
Philadelphia, PA 19131
Tel: (213) 477-6444

Kendall Gerdes, M.D. is board certified in both internal medicine and allergy/immunology. After five years of general practice, he learned about the approach of Theron Randolph and went to train with him. In private practice since 1979, Dr. Gerdes is currently President of the American Academy of Environmental Medicine.

1617 Vine St.
Denver, CO 80206
Tel: (303) 377-8837

William J. Goldwag, M.D. is the Medical Director of the Center for Preventive/Holistic Medicine located in Southern California, and is on the board of directors of the American Holistic Medical Association. He has been one of the pioneers in the use of chelation therapy and other nutritional and complementary medical therapies for the treatment of chronic health disorders.

7499 Cerritos Ave.
Stanton, CA 90680
Tel: (714) 827-5180

Philip Jay Hodes, Ed.D. has spent three decades learning about holistic health, detoxification and orthomolecular nutritional therapies to rectify as well as prevent various conditions. He is a researcher, writer, speaker, and educator, as well as a health care practitioner.

144 Keer Ave.
Newark, N.J. 07112-1915

Abram Hoffer, M.D., Ph.D. received his Ph.D. from the University of Minnesota and his M.D. from the University of Toronto. He was Director of Psychiatric Research for the Province of Saskatchewan from 1950 to 1967. In private practice since 1967 specializing in the treatment of schizophrenia and cancer, he helped introduce orthomolecular medicine, in which vitamins are used as a primary treatment modality.

2727 Quadra St., Suite 3-A
Victoria, B.C.
Canada V8T 4E5
Tel: (604) 386-8756

Richard A. Kunin, M.D. is a founder and past president of the Orthomolecular Medical Society. He is in private practice, specializing in orthomolecular ecology medicine, in San Francisco.

2698 Pacific Ave.
San Francisco, CA 94115
Tel: (415) 346-2500

Stephen Langer, M.D. practices preventive medicine in Berkeley, California, specializing in the treatment of chronic fatigue, among other illnesses. He is President of the American Nutritional Medical Association.

3031 Telegraph Ave., #230
Berkeley, CA 94705
Tel: (510) 548-7384

Warren M. Levin, M.D. is currently celebrating his 20th anniversary as an orthomolecular physician. He is board certified in family practice, environmental medicine, and chelation therapy.

> 24 W. 57th St., Suite 701
> New York, N.Y. 10019
> Tel: (212) 397-5900

Doris J. Rapp, M.D. is a board certified pediatric allergist and specialist in environmental medicine. She has written and presented her videos of children's responses to physicians and the public in many countries. Videotapes of patients' responses to treatment can be obtained by calling 1-800-787-8780.

> 2757 Elmwood Ave.
> Buffalo, N.Y. 14217
> Tel: (716) 875-0398 or 875-5578

Michael B. Schachter, M.D. is a graduate of Columbia University's College of Physicians and Surgeons and a board certified psychiatrist. He has been practicing orthomolecular medicine and psychiatry since 1974. Dr. Schachter directs a health care facility in Suffern, New York, using nutritional medicine, chelation therapy, homeopathy and other complementary treatment methods.

> 2 Executive Blvd., Suite 202
> Suffern, N.Y. 10901
> Tel: (914) 368-4700

Priscilla Anne Slagle, M.D. has private practices in Los Angeles and Palm Springs. Specializing in nutritional medicine and psychiatry, she treats most illnesses from the perspective of diet change, nutritional supplementation and natural hormones as needed.

16542 Ventura Blvd., Suite 306
Encino, CA 91436
Tel: (310) 826-0175

Lendon H. Smith, M.D. is a graduate of the University of Oregon Medical School who practiced psychiatry in the U.S. Army from 1947 to 1949, then returned to civilian life in general practice/ pediatrics from 1951 to 1975, and has specialized in nutrition-based therapies since 1975. He is the author of thirteen books, including *Feed Your Kids Right*, *Feed Yourself Right*, and *Feed Your Body Right*.

950 S.W. 21st Ave., Apt. #902
Portland, OR 97205-1517
Tel: (503) 222-2525

Allan N. Spreen, M.D. is a general practitioner in Jacksonville, Florida, with a specialization in nutrition-based medicine.

Walt Stoll, M.D., A.B.F.P. is a board certified family practitioner with more than 30 years experience, the last seventeen of them as a holistic physician. During those seventeen years he has combined his traditional Western (allopathic) training with fifteen other healing philosophies, practiced by trained professionals in his Lexington, Kentucky, Holistic Medical Centre. On November 17, 1994, after 14 years of harassment by the Kentucky Medical Licensing Board, his license to practice medicine was revoked.

415 South Bonita Ave.
Panama City, FL 32401-3963
Tel: (904) 747-8669; fax: (904) 769-1436

Ricardo B. Tan, M.D. practices holistic and preventive medicine, including nutrition-based modalities, chelation therapy, acupuncture, sclerotherapy, and homeopathy.

> 3220 North Freeway
> Ft. Worth, TX 76111
> Tel: (817) 626-1993

Aubrey M. Worrell, Jr., M.D. is a board certified allergist/immunologist with special interests in clinical ecology, environmental medicine, and nutrition.

> 3900 Hickory St.
> Pine Bluff, AR 71603-6352
> Tel: (501) 535-8200

Ray C. Wunderlich, Jr., M.D. is a graduate of Columbia University's College of Physicians and Surgeons. He practices nutritional and preventive medicine.

> 666 6th St. South
> St. Petersburg, FL 33701-4845
> Tel: (813) 822-3612

José A. Yaryura-Tobias, M.D. is Medical Director at the Institute for Bio-Behavioral Therapy and Research. He has worked extensively on OCD and schizophrenia, and is a Visiting Professor at the University of Cuyo in Argentina.

> 935 Northern Blvd.
> Great Neck, N.Y. 11021
> Tel: (516) 487-7116

Garry M. Vickar, M.D., F.R.C.P. (C.) is a psychiatrist who specializes in acutely ill patients. With an active full-time private practice, Dr. Vickar is board certified in both the U.S. and Canada. He is Chief of the Department of Psychiatry and Medical Director of the Schizophrenia Treatment and Education Programs[sm] at Christian Hospitals and Chairman of the Mental Health Committee of the St. Louis Metropolitan Medical Society. He is also a fellow of the Academy of Orthomolecular Psychiatry, and past Chairman of their scientific meetings.

1245 Graham Rd., Suite 506
St. Louis, MO 63031
Tel: (314) 837-4900; fax: (314) 837-5646

Alfred V. Zamm, M.D. is a diplomate of both the American Board of Dermatology and the American Board of Environmental Medicine. In addition to his private practice based in Kingston, New York, he is a consultant to five hospitals in the Hudson Valley.

111 Maiden Lane
Kingston, N.Y. 12401-4597
Tel: (914) 338-7766

INDEX

AA. *See* Alcoholic's Anonymous

Academy of Environmental
Medicine. *See* American
Academy of Environmental
Medicine

acupressure, 52

acupuncture, 20, 52

adhesives, 208, 210

adrenal gland, 111, 112, 129

adrenaline, 86, 146

aggression, in children, 177-182
causes of, 177-178
environmental toxicity and,
177-178
personal account of, 180-182
scientific abstracts on,
232-234
symptoms of, 178-179
treatment of, 179-180

agoraphobia, 24

AIDS, 20, 61

air purifiers, 180

Alcoholics Anonymous, 15, 76,
84

alcoholism, vii, viii, 13-16, 10,
35-36, 43, 51-52, 75-76, 113,
151-152, 223
causes of, 13-14
depression and, 35-36, 43,
151-152
personal account of, 15-16
schizophrenia and, 75-76,
151-152
scientific abstracts on,
234-251
sugar addiction and, 13
treatment of, 14-15
tryptophan and, 10

allergies, 8, 38, 45, 71, 105, 106,
117, 162, 178, 179-180,
205-219
children and, 205-219

allergy extract, 209

allergy testing, 6, 8, 199, 209
provocation/neutralization
method of, 209

aluminum toxicity, 18, 22, 68,
155, 165, 196

Alzheimer's Disease, 17-23, 155
aluminum exposure and, 18,
22, 155
chelation therapy and, 19
heavy metals and, 19, 22
homeopathic remedies and,
19-20
magnesium and, 21
scientific abstracts on,
151-258
senile dementia and, 21-22
treatment of, 18-22

AMA. *See* American Medical
Association

American Academy of
Environmental Medicine,
150, 197

American Medical Association, 8

amino acids , 24-25, 39, 51, 58,
61, 69, 83, 110, 114, 115, 116,
199

amphetamines, 36-37

animal feed, 156

anorexia, 48-50
cognitive therapy and, 49-50
scientific abstracts on, 258
treatment of, 40-50
zinc deficiency and, 48-49

Anti-Aging Plan, The, 17

antibiotics, 93, 118, 188, 195,
199
candida and, 199

antidepressants, 70, 131

antihistamine, 206

anxiety disorders, 3, 24-27, 53,
83, 114, 126, 131-135, 162
amino acids and, 24-25, 114
calcium and, 3